DIABETES

TO

WHOLENESS

A Natural and Spiritual Approach to

Disease Prevention & Healing!

Beth M. Ley, Ph.D.

BL Publications

Detroit Lakes, MN

BL Publications, Detroit Lakes, MN
For orders call 1-877-BOOKS11, also see www.blpbooks.com
email: blpub@tekstar.com

Library of Congress Cataloging-in-Publication Data
Ley, Beth M., 1964-
Diabetes to wholeness: a natural and spiritual approach to disease prevention & healing! / Beth M. Ley.
 p. ; cm.
Includes bibliographical references and index.
ISBN 1-890766-23-2
1. Non-insulin-dependent diabetes--Popular works. 2. Non-insulin-dependent diabetes--Alternative treatment. 3. Non-insulin-dependent diabetes--Religious aspects--Christianity. [DNLM: 1. Diabetes Mellitus--diet therapy--Popular Works. 2. Holistic Health--Popular Works. 3. Religion and Medicine--Popular Works. WK 818 L681d 2002] I. Title.
RC662.18 .L49 2002
616.4'62--dc21
                                        2002005146

Printed in the United States of America

This book is not intended as medical advice. Its purpose is solely educational. Please consult your healthcare professional for all health problems.

All scriptures are taken from The King James Version of the Holy Bible unless otherwise stated.

Credits: Cover Design: BL Publications
Proofreading: Karen Schultz

> ***Use food as your medicine and medicine as your food.*** Hippocrates
>
> ***The doctor of the future will give no medicine, but will interest his patients in the care of the human frame, in diet, and in the cause and prevention of disease.*** Thomas Edison

Table of Contents

YOU NEED TO KNOW...
THE HEALTH MESSAGE

Do you not know that you are God's temple and that God's Spirit dwells in you? If anyone destroys God's temple, God will destroy him. For God's temple is holy, and that temple you are. (*1 Corinthians 3:16-17 RSV*)

So, whether you eat or drink, or whatever you do, do all to the glory of God.
(*1 Corinthians 10:31 RSV*)

Introduction

There is something seriously wrong with the way most of society views health problems. Most people are looking for a quick cure for whatever ails them, but that will be of little "cost" to them. We don't want to change our eating habits, our thinking, or our lifestyle. Most prefer to take a pill to mask symptoms and continue on doing whatever pleases us. We don't realize the true (physical and emotional) cost of side effects and continued pain and suffering while the root of the problem remains. While the medical community continues in its attempt to obtain disease management, largely through drugs, what I am interested in is **complete freedom from disease and disease prevention!**

Pharmaceuticals (prescription and over-the-counter) in most cases work by force, which is accompanied by side effects, and only mask symptoms of a health problem. They can help you lower your cholesterol levels – but have no effect on the root problem that is causing your cholesterol levels to be elevated in the first place. Curing your health problem, by the way, is not the goal of the pharmaceutical companies as it would not be financially of benefit to them. They make more money if you have to take the drug every day for the rest of your life.

In contrast, a diet based on whole foods and dietary supplements encourage the body to do what it was designed to do, which is heal itself – and almost never have side effects.

In counseling at the Wellness Center, I must address "wellness" from all aspects (body, soul and spirit) to actually see improvements and sometimes complete healing of health problems. Improving the diet and taking supplements *alone* does not always work. Prayer *alone* does not always work. Making lifestyle, relationship and attitude changes (correcting unforgiveness, stress, anxiety etc.) *alone* does not always work. But, a combination of *all of these* **almost always works.**

Remember, healing is a process. While God is fully capable of instant healing (which we do occasionally see), your health problems usually do not come upon you overnight, but have been a degenerative process. In the same manner, healing is progressional. Once you get going in the right direction, God will bless you in healing of both emotional and physical areas of your life. God is into restoration! He wants to restore His people!

So many people claim to be "saved" and yet do not allow Christ to do **all** of what He came to do in their lives. *The Spirit of the Lord [is] upon me, because he hath anointed me to preach the gospel to the poor; he hath sent me to* **heal the brokenhearted**, *to preach* **deliverance to the captives**, *and* **recovering of sight to the blind**, *to* **set at liberty them that are bruised**. (Luke 4:18)

I am not interested in seeing mere improvements in symptoms, I want to see a complete change of **bondage to freedom** in your lives! This freedom does not come without cost, and it does not come without a degree of responsibility. Freedom is conditional upon your obedience to **all** that God requires (body, soul and spirit). This is no easy task. But **it is possible** and many do enjoy this life of freedom! (Myself included, despite the many years of health challenges I experienced!)

The health problem focused upon in this book is diabetes. My concerns for diabetes largely stem from the increased number of adults and especially <u>children</u> developing adult-onset diabetes, and the younger and younger age this is occurring. Because the cause of this type of diabetes is largely dietary, this clearly tells me we are not feeding our children correctly. This type of diabetes was named **adult**-onset because it was in adulthood (usually age 50, 60 or 70), when it would appear. The dietary habits that used to take 50 or 60 years to wear out the body (resulting in Type II diabetes), we now can accomplish in only 12 or 15 years. This is very sad, but, it is no shock if one closely examines the eating habits popular today. Refined foods are destroying our health. Marketing experts have most of the population convinced that buying these garbage foods with their colorful packaging, toys inside the box, and convenience is more important than our health. We need to take control over our eating habits, control over our lives and start living the life free of the bondage of disease that God has planned for us!

God is He *who forgiveth all thine iniquities; who healeth all thy diseases.* (Psalms 103:3)

This book addresses the healing and prevention of diabetes through all three aspects of wellness, the body, soul and spirit. By examining and correcting your health problems from all three aspects, you too can be whole!

Diabetes

Diabetes mellitus affects nearly 16 million people in the United States. By the year 2010, the projected number is 22 million. The direct and indirect cost of diabetes mellitus is now $40 billion per year. It is the third leading cause of death in the United States after heart disease and cancer.

Diabetes insipidus, a less common condition, refers to a hormonal imbalance that affects the kidneys.

Diabetes mellitus is associated with abnormally high levels of sugar (glucose) in the blood. It is characterized by a decreased ability, or complete inability, of the body to utilize carbohydrates as fuel for our cells. Sugar levels in the blood normally increase after eating carbohydrates, which break down into sugar (glucose). In healthy individuals, blood glucose levels are tightly controlled by insulin, a hormone produced by the pancreas. Insulin works to lower the blood glucose level in the blood by escorting glucose into our cells to be burned for energy. However, in diabetics, the absence of insulin, the insufficient production of insulin, or the resistance of the cells to insulin causes elevated sugar levels in the blood (hyperglycemia).

An elevated glucose level in the blood is very stressful to the body. It can damage blood vessels and nerves, impair circulation, and eventually lead to numerous complications such as blindness, kidney failure and nerve damage. Diabetes is also an important factor in accelerating the hardening and narrowing of the arteries (atherosclerosis), stroke, coronary heart diseases and other blood vessel diseases in the body.

Unable to use glucose for energy, the body begins to burn fat and proteins (muscle). Symptoms include fatigue, irritability, excessive thirst, increased urination, and in Type I diabetics, weight loss (despite increased hunger and food intake).

There are two kinds of diabetes mellitus: Type I and Type II.

Type I (insulin-dependent diabetes or IDDM) is much less common than Type II diabetes, affecting about 10% of all those who have diabetes. It is also known as juvenile-onset diabetes, because it often begins in children or young adults. In Type I diabetes, the pancreas is unable to produce insulin, and insulin medication is relied upon for survival. This type of diabetes can only be controlled by taking insulin (through injection or a pump). Diet is also very important to help control blood sugar.

Type I diabetes is an autoimmune condition in which the body attacks its own cells of the pancreas. Normally, the immune system is designed to protect the body against foreign invaders and infections. In autoimmune diseases, the immune system mistakenly manufactures antibodies that are directed against and cause damage to one's own body tissues. There is a genetically inherited tendency to develop these abnormal antibodies in IDDM.

Type II (non-insulin-dependent diabetes or NIDD) is much more prevalent than Type I. In Type II diabetes, the pancreas produces insulin but the cells in the body cannot use it effectively, resulting in insulin resistance. After several years, insulin production decreases, glucose builds up in the blood, and the body cannot make efficient use of its main source of fuel, glucose. Ineffective glucose burning creates serious health problems such as heart disease, neuropathy and blindness.

Syndrome X is a condition which refers to a group of health problems associated with insulin resistance. Over time, left untreated, this can progress to Type II diabetes.

Type II diabetes is also known as adult-onset diabetes, because it usually occurs in older adults and can be managed with a careful diet, exercise and careful self-monitoring. It is almost 100% preventable with a proper whole foods diet that avoids processed foods. Type II diabetes is linked to:

- Being overweight

- African American, Native American or Hispanic heritage

- A diet high in processed foods such as sugar and low in fiber and complex carbohydrates

- A family history of diabetes.

Some Type II diabetics do not produce adequate amounts of insulin. The pancreas may be inefficient or slow to release the needed insulin in response to increased glucose levels. Finally, the liver continues to produce glucose despite elevated glucose levels.

Diabetes can also occur transiently during pregnancy, probably related to the stress on the body at that time.

Refined Diet Causing Type II Diabetes Sooner

A disturbing change is that Type II diabetes, which previously was only rarely seen in young individuals, is now occurring more and more frequently in young children. As children continue to eat a highly refined diet and overeat and not exercise, adult-onset diabetes is appearing in overweight children at alarming rates. We are consuming 30% more refined foods than we did in 1970. This is clearly having a detrimental effect not only upon our health, but upon our children's health.

Because refined foods tend to be less filling and less satisfying (since most of the fiber and nutrients are lost), overeating of these foods is an added problem that greatly stresses the body.

Refined foods do not satisfy our nutritional needs and actually create nutritional deficiencies, which get worse with the more refined foods that are eaten. Certain nutrients (lost in refining and processing) are needed by the body to metabolize what is consumed. When we eat whole, natural foods (the way God made them), the nutrients (B vitamins, minerals, enzymes, etc.) we need to digest them are largely provided in the food.

Nutritional deficiencies are created by a diet high in refined foods. Adequate levels of minerals such as magnesium, calcium, potassium, zinc, chromium, and vanadium, for example, have great importance for proper use of insulin in the body. Amino acids, including L-carnitine, taurine, and L-arginine, also play a role in the proper use of insulin by cells. Antioxidants levels are also important as it is known that antioxidant nutrients such as glutathione, CoQ10, and lipoic acid, have therapeutic potential to improve insulin resistance.

This refined diet is also affecting older generations resulting in the increased incidence of diabetes in all age groups. In 1997, the federal government recommended that all adults be tested for diabetes before age 45. That same year, the American Diabetes Association (ADA) lowered the fasting plasma glucose (FPG) value in diagnosing diabetics from 140 mg./dl. or higher to a standard FPG value of 126 mg./dl. A FPG of 126 mg./dl. or higher is associated with an increased risk of diabetes complications affecting the eyes, nerves and kidneys.

Syndrome X: *Precursor to Type II diabetes*
Do you frequently experience:

- Fatigue, especially after eating?
- Difficulty concentrating, fuzzy thinking?
- Irritability or anger?
- Cravings for refined carbohydrates such as pasta, bread, crackers, baked goods, etc.?
- Tendency to binge on sweets and carbohydrate foods?
- Shakiness if you do not eat regular meals?
- Weight gain and difficulty losing it?
- Are 10 or more pounds overweight?
- In men, have a "pot belly" or "love handles"?
- In women, carry fat in your abdominal region rather than thighs and hips?
- Elevated cholesterol (above 240 mg./dl.) or take medication to lower your cholesterol?
- Elevated triglycerides (above 160 mg./dl.)?
- Have high blood pressure (above 140/90) or take medication to lower your blood pressure?
- Unexplained thirst and/or need to urinate frequently?

The more "yes" answers you have to these questions indicates a more serious condition of Syndrome X and the more likely you are to developing or already having Type II diabetes.

Glucose Regulation

The body was incredibly designed to be self regulating. The scientific community calls this process homeostasis (*homeo* meaning same, *stasis* meaning change). This means that the body is always making adjustments in order to keep it self the same (in balance). This is done through various hormones, neurotransmitters and a complicated biofeedback system. It is all done automatically, involving no thought on our part. When we eat, for example, we do not have to tell our salivary glands or our pancreas to release digestive enzymes to begin breaking the food down.

This is indeed a blessing, but it can also be a curse if the body is misused. For example, if our diet is lacking in certain minerals such as calcium or phosphorous, and blood levels become low, the body sends message and the needed minerals will be obtained from the body's mineral storage units – the bones. If this dietary pattern continues, over time the bones will become mineral depleted, brittle, and prone to fractures. This is known as osteoporosis. This is a fairly well-known example, but there are hundreds of other medical problems associated with nutritional deficiencies. Less well-known examples include:

- A chromium (a trace mineral) deficiency can cause insulin resistance, diabetes, weight gain, etc.

- An Omega-3 (an essential fatty acid) deficiency can cause prostaglandin imbalances causing inflammatory disorders such as arthritis, psoriasis, eczema, dermatitis, allergies, etc.

- A folic acid (a B vitamin) deficiency can cause hair to turn gray, gastrointestinal disturbances, lesions at the corner of the mouth, and anemia that is not corrected by iron supplementation. Folic acid is needed to form red blood cells.

Glucose or "blood sugar" is the simplest form of all carbohydrates and is the molecule that the body's cells burn to fuel all life processes. Complex carbohydrates (also known as starches which includes bread, rice, pasta, potatoes, etc.) contain long chains of glucose molecules bound together that must be broken down by the digestive tract through various enzymes. Simple carbohydrates contain shorter chains of glucose molecules such as fructose (fruit sugar), dextrose (from corn) or glucose (table sugar) which is already broken down and therefore, is very quickly absorbed into the blood stream.

Glucose is absolutely essential to life, but it must circulate throughout the body in a well-maintained balance for proper health. The main problem in diabetes is too much blood sugar (too little also endangers health).

After meals, food is digested in the stomach and the intestines. The glucose from digested carbohydrate foods is absorbed by the intestinal cells into the bloodstream and is carried by blood to all the cells in the body to be burned. However, glucose cannot enter the cells alone. It requires assistance from insulin (and chromium) to

> **The following lead to elevated blood sugar levels and diabetes mellitus:**
>
> - Complete lack of insulin
> - Insufficient production of insulin
> - Production of defective insulin
> - Inability of cells to use insulin (insulin resistance) most often caused by nutritional deficiencies caused by a diet high in refined foods.

penetrate the cell walls. Without insulin, cells become starved of glucose energy despite the presence of abundant glucose in the blood. Some of the abundant, unutilized glucose is wastefully excreted in the urine (hence the term *sweet urine*) and the rest is converted into glycogen, a complex form of glucose that is stored in the liver and and muscle tissues to be used later as energy.

Insulin, produced by the pancreas, helps glucose enter the cells to regulate the level of glucose in the blood. When blood glucose levels are lowered, the insulin release is turned off. In normal individuals, such a regulatory system helps to keep blood glucose levels in a tightly controlled range.

In diabetics, the insulin is either missing (as in Type I diabetes), or insulin regulation is defective and insufficient (as in Type II diabetes). Both cause elevated levels of blood glucose (hyperglycemia).

Unstable glucose levels can result from a number of reasons, most of them dietary, which means we are in control. Emotional factors such as stress also play a role, but we are also in control of our emotions. If we live our life according to our circumstances, we are living in bondage and need be freed from that.

Elevated blood glucose levels create problems:

- Excess glucose that cannot be burned is converted to glycogen in the liver, which is stored as fat and results in weight gain.

- Triglyceride levels increase in the blood. (Triglycerides are a form of fats in the blood stream formed from glucose.)

- Free radical activity increases causing tissue damage (this is discussed in detail later) and numerous complications associated with diabetes.

- Creates a state of high insulin levels in the blood, leading to weight gain and eventually insulin resistance, more weight gain, and eventually, most likely, Type II diabetes.

Insulin and Weight Gain

Insulin is a hormone produced and secreted by the beta cells of the pancreas following the consumption of carbohydrates to maintain the proper balance of glucose in the blood stream. This hormone also controls our metabolism. It brings glucose, amino acids and free fatty acids into our cells where potential energy is stored as fat and glycogen to be used later. Insulin promotes the storage of all food groups and therefore, weight gain, if those calories are not burned. The stored calories are available for use as energy later in fasting or between meals. When insulin levels drop (between meals as blood glucose levels drop) stored fats and stored sugar (glycogen) are then used as energy sources.

Obese individuals have elevated insulin levels continually. Weight gain and obesity are the first problems to occur with insulin resistance. Normally, a small amount of insulin will adequate lower glucose levels, but more in required in insulin resistant individuals. Insulin in the blood stream causes fat to be stored.The more insulin present, the more fat is stored.

An obese individual may be on their way to the development of Type II diabetes if the insulin-resistance problem is not taken care of. The pancreas may become exhausted from constant stimulation by glucose and eventually fail.

Normally, after eating, insulin is released and during fasting another pancreatic hormone, glucagon is released when blood sugar levels fall too low. This mobilizes stored fat into glucose, which raises the blood sugar level back to normal.

The good news is that 50% or more of insulin resistance can be reduced or reversed through dietary changes! There are many things we can do to help stabilize blood glucose and insulin levels. Good dietary habits are important for a number of reasons. Processing and refining of foods changes the way they act in the body after we eat them – and not in a good way. The nutritional deficiencies resulting from eating processed foods interfere with proper carbohydrate digestion, functioning of insulin, cellular integrity and other details to be discussed later.

Chromium, a trace mineral, is naturally present in foods that contain carbohydrates (sugars), but it is one of the many nutrients lost in the refining process. Over 90%

of the chromium and other nutrients are lost in the processing of whole wheat to white flour or of sugar cane or sugar beets to white sugar. Chromium acts as the door opener for the cells to allow glucose to enter and to be burned. Without adequate chromium, the cells will not allow the glucose in to be burned no matter how much insulin is present.

Other nutrients lost (such as B vitamins and other minerals) are required for proper digestion. Without them, problems such as fluctuating glucose levels and weight gain result.

Fiber is also lost in the refining process. This speeds up the absorption of sugars into the bloodstream, causing glucose levels to rise more quickly, creating an unnecessary burden upon the pancreas.

Basic Goals for Type I and Type II Diabetics

- Prevent erratic blood glucose levels by avoiding processed foods, especially refined carbohydrates.

- Keep blood lipids low to prevent cardiovascular disease by avoiding saturated fats and sugar.

- Nourish the body with **whole foods** in their natural form. A healthy, high-fiber, low-fat diet, with added supplements (especially antioxidants and others discussed in this book) can help to prevent some diabetic complications.

- Maintain regular moderate exercise.

- For Type II diabetics, weight loss may also treat the disease. Weight control is an important element of diabetes self-care.

Nutritional Support

A whole-food, low-fat diet rich in fiber and complex carbohydrates lowers your diabetes risk. In addition, several minerals and vitamins taken as supplements have been found to be helpful in staving off or controlling this condition.

Zinc and chromium are well known as important trace elements for diabetics as cofactors for proper insulin production and use. Recently, some essential trace elements such as vanadium and selenium were observed to have several physiological insulin-like effects. Chromium, manganese, vanadium, and selenium have a favorable effect on carbohydrate metabolism. (Kimura)

These important nutrients are lost in the processing of foods, yet are crucial for proper digestion by the body.

Chromium

This essential trace mineral helps maximize insulin's effectiveness in controlling blood sugar levels and may help prevent diabetes. Insulin uses chromium as a cofactor in unlocking the cell membrane, allowing glucose to enter the cell. The mineral has a significant amount of research demonstrating its benefits in improving blood sugar control in Type I and II diabetics. Chromium also lowers cholesterol and aids in fat loss without impacting lean body mass.

Suboptimal dietary intake of chromium is associated with increased risk factors associated with diabetes and cardiovascular diseases. Research demonstrates chromium improves glucose and related variables in subjects with glucose intolerance and Type I and II gestational and steroid-induced diabetes.

Chromium works by increasing insulin binding to cells, and increases active insulin receptors (kinase) leading to increased insulin sensitivity. (Anderson, RA)

Therapeutic levels are required (400-1,000 mcg. daily): Severe neuropathy and glucose intolerance of a patient receiving nutrients through a feeding rube, who was receiving currently recommended levels of chromium, were reversed by additional supplemental chromium. (Anderson, RA)

Scientists from China and the United States Department of Agriculture showed that Type II diabetics who took large doses of chromium (1,000 mcg. daily) had glucose and insulin levels close to normal as the chromium helped stabilize blood sugar levels.

Another study showed that insulin sensitivity greatly increased in obese individuals at high risk of developing Type II diabetes after taking 1,000 mcg. chromium for eight months. Chromium also helps reduce body fat while maintaining lean muscle tissue. Another study had similar results at 400 mcg. daily. Other studies show dosages at 100 mcg. daily are too low to be effective. More than 100 scientific papers have cited chromium, at the proper dosage, to be safe and effective to help maintain healthy blood sugar levels.

The recommended therapeutic daily intake of chromium is 400-600 mcg. Because chromium makes the insulin that you have (either naturally produced or through medication) work better, you need to be careful to avoid low blood sugar until your body adjusts. Be sure to check your glucose levels frequently so you can see how it is affecting you. You may need to adjust your medication if you are on any.

Intake recommended for nondiabetics is 200 mcg. daily. Watch for products containing chromium chloride, as this is a less absorbable form. You may not absorb adequate amounts from this form.

Foods high in chromium include:

Brewer's yeast	Liver	Wheat germ
Cracked wheat	Corn meal	Buckwheat
Molasses	Apples	Prunes
Clams	Shrimp	Lobster
Mushrooms	Whole grains	

Vanadium

Vanadium is a trace mineral that seems to enhance insulin action in diabetics, according to several studies. In one study, people with Type II diabetes who took 50 mcg. of vanadium sulfate twice a day for four weeks had a 20% decrease in fasting blood sugar levels. Vanadium also has an insulin-like effect, and it decreases blood sugar levels. If people take supplemental vanadium, they may need less chromium. One might start on five mcg. of vanadyl sulfate three times a day with meals, then cut back to five mcg. once a day as blood sugar levels move into a normal range. The dosage may need to be

21

regulated with your doctor's supervision.

Not everyone does well on this mineral. Some people say they feel more clear-headed, their blood sugar is stabilized, and they feel great. Others, however, feel just the opposite: light-headed, spacey and shaky. If you experience these reactions, you should stop taking vanadium.

The safety of long-term use has not been demonstrated, and results of some animal studies suggest concern about long-term toxicity.

There's also the possibility of stomach upset. In one study, six of eight people reported diarrhea, abdominal cramps, gas, and nausea the first week they took vanadium. After that, however, their symptoms stopped.

Magnesium

Low magnesium levels are associated with glucose intolerance, a prediabetic condition. In a study of elderly people, magnesium supplements improved glucose handling. Involved in several aspects of carbohydrate metabolism, magnesium helps release insulin and transport sugar. Magnesium helps vitamin B6 get inside cells, where both the mineral and the vitamin play central roles in energy production. Some people with diabetes have low levels of magnesium, and there's some evidence that getting enough may help prevent complications such as damage to the retina of the eye and heart disease.

Magnesium-rich foods include: beans, whole grains, leafy greens, tofu, nuts and seeds.

The recommended supplemental intake is 500-800 mg. daily. Magnesium gluconate or citrate are good absorbable supplemental forms.

Zinc

Some researchers believe that a lack of zinc makes you more prone to diabetes. Zinc is a vital constituent of your body's chemicals involved in insulin metabolism. Zinc also improves glucose tolerance in laboratory animals.

Zinc deficiency is commonly associated with insulin resistance and Type II diabetes. (Simon, Kelly) Zinc is plentiful in the healthy pancreas, where insulin is manufactured, and is a constituent of insulin.

One large cross-sectional survey revealed that lower consumption of dietary zinc and low serum zinc levels were associated with an increased prevalence of diabetes, coronary artery disease, and several of their associated risk factors, including high blood pressure, elevated triglycerides, and insulin resistance in urban individuals. (Singh)

Another study provided evidence that a low groundwater content of zinc (reflecting long-term deficiency through less than optimal drinking water) is associated with development of juvenile-onset diabetes. A high groundwater concentration of zinc was associated with a significant decrease in risk of diabetes development. (Haglund)

Zinc is essential for proper development of reproductive organs and health of the prostate gland. It is also necessary for proper B vitamin utilization, digestion, healing, and the synthesis of nucleic acid. Extensive zinc depletion can have serious effects on the immune system especially when fighting against degenerative diseases. A zinc deficiency is also a factor in stress, fatigue, loss of taste or smell, and decreased alertness. At least 25 enzymes are dependent on zinc.

Zinc is found in protein foods such as meat, fish, and eggs, unprocessed whole grains, brewer's yeast, wheat bran and germ, mushrooms, black-eyed peas and pumpkin seeds.

Recommended supplemental intake is 25-50 mg. daily.

Diabetics tend to be deficient in certain minerals, including magnesium, manganese, chromium and zinc. (Kruse-Jarres)
In addition to poor diet, this is possibly a side effect of medications.

B-Complex Vitamins

B-complex vitamins are essential for your body to convert sugar and starches to energy, a chemical process called carbohydrate metabolism. A shortage of any one of them can cause problems. Vitamin B6 deficiency has been linked to glucose intolerance, which is an abnormally high rise in blood sugar after eating.

B vitamin shortages can also lead to nerve damage in the hands and feet. Some studies indicate that people with diabetes develop less of the numbness and tingling associated with diabetes-related nerve damage if they take supplemental B vitamins.

Diabetics tend to use up their B vitamins more quickly than non-diabetics. Also, poorly controlled diabetes causes these nutrients to be excreted in the urine.

One particular B vitamin, a form of niacin known as niacinamide, may actually help prevent Type I diabetes from developing in high-risk individuals. B complex supplementation is recommended.

Antioxidants

The normal metabolism of glucose (from the carbohydrate foods we eat) in the body generates a large number of harmful byproducts called free radicals or oxidants. These free radicals oxidize or damage other cells, creating a cascade of harmful molecules. Elevated blood sugar causes a number of serious problems. Normal glucose levels for a diabetic (180-250 mg./dl.) are almost twice the normal range (70-120 mg./dl.) for non-diabetics.

Free radicals are highly reactive molecules that are missing an electron, which normally exist in pairs. Therefore, they "steal" electrons from other healthy molecules, thereby creating another free radical.

Every time a free radical causes the transfer of an electron, it weakens the molecule and, eventually, tissue damage results. Free radicals cause protein damage as the nonenzymatic joining of sugar to protein forms destructive oxygen radicals. The process of forming sugar-damaged proteins is called **glycation**, which can be compared to the browning reaction of sliced apples.

Blood sugar (glucose) and some other sugars react spontaneously with collagen, a major protein found in skin, blood vessels, and connective tissue, and other proteins to form cross-linked, sugar-damaged proteins.

When these are formed, additional free radicals are released as well. (Tritschler)

In diabetics, damage from these reactions is magnified because of the elevated sugar levels. As blood sugar levels rise and remain elevated, the rate at which free radicals are formed and sugar-damaged proteins are formed increases accordingly.

Blood Sugar, Aging, Insulin Resistance and Disease

The spontaneous reaction of sugar with tissue proteins such as collagen and myelin is responsible for accelerated tissue aging in diabetics, is believed responsible for kidney damage, and is also involved in the atherosclerosis process. These are both common complications of diabetes. Dr. Anthony Cerami observed that glycation reactions also play a role in the normal aging of tissue. Recent studies show that diabetics as well as aging animals do indeed have increased concentrations of damaged proteins in their collagen.

As we age, our average blood sugar level tends to rise. This is because our tissues become less sensitive to the actions of insulin (insulin resistance) as we get older.

The roles of oxygen- and sugar-damaged protein definitely explain many of the secondary aging effects and some of the primary aging process. Maintaining stable and optimal blood sugar levels throughout life should protect or slow down our tissues from aging.

Both free radical reduction and glycation reduction reduce the incidence of the aging diseases, including heart disease, cataracts, macular degeneration, arthritis and cancer. They are complimentary approaches that enhance each other's benefits. The protection against free radical damage is more efficient with both approaches than through the actions of either alone.

Some cellular damage caused by radicals can be repaired by enzymes. We actually produce some enzymes in the body for the sole purpose of repairing damage to cells caused by radicals and by high levels of blood sugar. However, adequate levels of antioxidants are needed to protect these enzymes from free radical damage as well.

Antioxidants

To combat the free radicals (oxidants) that we create (and also those we are exposed to in the environment through various toxins, pollution, cigarette smoke, etc.), the body uses antioxidants. Some of these are produced by the body, others come through the foods we eat or supplements we take. These include vitamins C and E, beta carotene, zinc, glutathione, lipoic acid, CoQ10 and and many botanical extracts such as ginkgo biloba and procyanidins (grapeseed extract). As long as the ratio of free radicals to antioxidants remains in balance, the damage resulting from the circulating free radicals will be minimized.

In diabetics, free radical levels are sky high and the level of antioxidants are very depressed. The long-term effects of elevated blood sugar levels is oxidative tissue damage (glycation). This is the cause of the diabetic complications such as cataracts, retinopathy, macular degeneration, stiffened arteries and heart tissue via damaged lipoproteins (LDL), and nerve destruction (polyneuropathy). High sugar levels can also result in osmotic changes and reduced blood volume, shock acidosis, coma and death.

Insulin-dependent diabetics also use up more

27

antioxidants such as vitamin C - increasing the risk for free radical damage. Antioxidants such as vitamins C and E, and lipoic acid may protect you from oxidative damage and even reduce your risk of diabetes, although this has not been conclusively proven.

Vitamin C

Vitamin C helps regulate blood sugar levels as it works with insulin. It also accelerates healing, is needed for bone and tooth formation, collagen production, prevention of common cold, digestion, red blood cell formation, shock and infection resistance, and is thought to contain cancer protection agents.

Good food sources include rose hips, citrus fruits, black currants, berries, broccoli, cabbage, cauliflower, persimmons, guavas, sweet potatoes and green bell peppers.

Vitamin E

Vitamin E improves the cardiovascular system in Type II diabetics.

Type II diabetes is associated with elevated oxidative stress and declines in antioxidant defense. The disease is also characterized by an imbalance in the ratio of cardiac sympathetic to parasympathetic tone. Antioxidants, vitamin E in particular, may have beneficial effects on the cardiac autonomic nervous system through a decline in oxidative stress. (Manzella)

Vitamin E also helps to lower blood sugar levels. Vitamin E is also an anticoagulant, alleviates fatigue, dilates blood vessels, reduces blood cholesterol, improves circulation, capillary formation and functioning of red blood cells, muscle, and other tissues, and protects essential fatty acids.

Good food sources include vegetable oils, whole grain cereals, wheat germ, lettuce, brussels sprouts, leafy greens, soybeans and eggs.

In diabetics, free radical levels are sky high and antioxidant levels are very depressed.

α-Lipoic Acid

Alpha lipoic acid (or lipoic acid) is probably the most important supplement that I recommend to diabetics. I have seen so many benefits that I am thoroughly convinced of its merits. For diabetics supplementing lipoic acid, many need to reduce their insulin intake because of its ability to increase the effectiveness of insulin. Long-term use of lipoic acid proves its protective effects against complications commonly seen among diabetics.

Lipoic acid is a powerful antioxidant found in the body and also in many foods such as potatoes, spinach, yams and carrots. Some studies show lipoic acid supplementation increases the uptake and utilization of glucose by over 50%. Studies on animals show lipoic acid can reduce diabetic nerve damage. Lipoic acid is effectively used therapeutically throughout Europe to treat and prevent complications of diabetes such as polyneuropathy and macular degeneration.

As an antioxidant, lipoic acid is 30 to 50 times more powerful than vitamins C or E.

Lipoic Acid Levels Lower in Diabetics

Individuals diagnosed with diabetes and many of the complications associated with diabetes such as polyneuropathy and atherosclerosis have been found to have lower levels of endogenous (produced in the body) lipoic acid. (Altnkirch, Piering) Because higher levels of free radical damage have been shown to be a characteristic of these conditions, there is great benefit in lipoic acid supplementation. Supplemental lipoic acid helps restore normal lipoic acid levels in the body, which are known to be low in diabetics.

Lipoic Acid Benefits Diabetes Type I and II

Lipoic acid has potential beneficial effects for both types of diabetes. Both human and animal studies show that lipoic acid enhances glucose utilization. Studies in obese individuals show lipoic acid treatment increased the uptake of glucose in the absence or presence of insulin in muscles by over 50%. (Henricksen) 1,000 mg. of lipoic acid administered intravenously to diabetics enhanced insulin-stimulated whole body glucose disposal by about 50%. (Jacob)

The various beneficial effects of lipoic acid for diabetics are believed to be involved in the regulation of insulin-stimulated glucose transport in to the cells (lowering insulin resistance). The effect may also be due to the protective antioxidant function of lipoic acid. (Packer)

Lipoic Acid Normalizes Blood Sugar Levels

Lipoic acid not only normalizes blood sugar levels in diabetics, it also protects against the damage responsible for diabetes in the first place. It has been successfully used in Germany for more than 30 years where it has reduced the secondary effects of diabetes, including damage to the retina, cataract formation, and nerve and heart damage, as well as increasing energy levels. Lipoic acid improves nerve blood flow, reduces oxidative stress, and improves distal nerve conduction in neuropathy.

Researchers have demonstrated the potential for the therapeutic use of lipoic acid against diabetes-induced complications. (Suzuki) A study at the University of California, Berkeley, also showed that this substance may play a role in the prevention of diabetic complications by inhibiting glycation and structural damage of proteins. (Kawabata, Hofmann)

Lipoic acid can terminate free radicals and thus reduce the oxidative stress that can damage the pancreas, cause cataracts, nerve damage, retinopathy and other side effects. Lipoic acid also reduces glycation, which otherwise can damage proteins, especially those of skin and blood vessels. Even more important to diabetics is that lipoic acid, by virtue of its ability to normalize blood sugar levels and the entire pathway for conversion of sugar into energy, allows the nerves to heal and recover. Pain is reduced and normal feeling is restored.

Lipoic acid increases glucose transport by stimulating the glucose transporters to move from the cell interior to the membrane. This action is independent of insulin transport. This restoration of normal blood sugar levels in turn increases the number of glucose transporters in the membranes of muscle cells. This is a very desirable cycle.

Lipoic acid supplementation (300-600 mg. per day, taken in two to three divided doses) significantly lowers blood sugar, sorbitol, serum pyruvate and acetoacetate levels while increasing glycogen (stored energy compound for muscles) in muscles and the liver. At the same time, there is an increase in blood sugar utilization by muscle tissues and a reduction in liver glucose output.

Glutathione, Cysteine Help Normalize Glucose

Lipoic acid also benefits levels of other antioxidants including glutathione and cysteine. Both of these amino acids play a critical role in blood sugar regulation.

In Germany, where lipoic acid is currently used as a treatment for diabetic polyneuropathy, researchers made a profound discovery in their efforts to demonstrate the ability of lipoic acid to enhance glucose utilization. As insulin resistance of skeletal muscle glucose uptake is a prominent feature of Type II diabetes, these interventions to improve insulin sensitivity could be of tremendous benefit.

The study involved 13 patients who received 1,000 mg. lipoic acid and the controls who did not. Both groups were comparable in age, body-mass index, and duration of diabetes and had a similar baseline of insulin resistance. Lipoic acid proved beneficial as it significantly increases insulin-stimulated glucose disposal from the blood. The metabolic clearance rate for glucose rose by about 50% in those supplementing lipoic acid, whereas the control group did not show any significant change. The mode of action of lipoic acid on glucose is not yet completely clear. (Jacob)

CAUTION: Because of the effects of lipoic acid supplementation on diabetics, modification of insulin or oral antidiabetic intake may be required to prevent hypoglycemic states. Close monitoring of blood glucose levels is required.

Lipoic Acid Improves Nerve Blood Flow, Regenerates Nerves, Reverses Polyneuropathy

Reduced nerve blood flow due to oxidative stress from elevated glucose levels is a serious problem among diabetics and is so serious that gangrene and amputation of limbs can be the result. Lipoic acid improves nerve blood flow, reduces oxidative stress, and improves distal nerve conduction in diabetic neuropathy.

Coenzyme Q-10 (CoQ10)

This enzyme/antioxidant is involved in the metabolic activity of all cells in the body. Some tissues in the body, such as the heart and pancreas, have higher concentrations than other tissues, signifying its importance to the health of these particular organs. CoQ10 has also demonstrated a protective effect on the beta islet function in the pancreas. These cells are highly susceptible to free radical damage. (Salonen) Supplemental CoQ10 and other antioxidants may help prevent some of this damage.

A number of researchers have demonstrated that diabetics have depressed levels of CoQ10, especially insulin-dependent diabetics. (McDonnell, Anderson) Another reason to supplement CoQ10 is to help maintain heart health. Research also shows that diabetic individuals with very low CoQ10 levels are extremely vulnerable to death from congestive heart failure. (Anderson)

A significant number of adult-onset diabetics (Type II) may have mitochondrial defects in the pancreas resulting in defective secretion of insulin. An enzyme (called glycerol-3-phosphate dehydrogenase or G3PD) that signals the pancreas to release insulin is underexpressed in the beta cells of Type II diabetics. Suboptimal tissue levels of CoQ10 could be expected to further impair G3PD activity. Clinical reports from Japan suggest that supplemental CoQ10 may often improve beta-cell function and glycemic control in Type II diabetics. (McCarty)

Researchers examining the effects of CoQ10 treatment on insulin secretory response found it to be beneficial. The 28 patients were treated daily with 150 mg. of CoQ10 orally for three years. Those in the CoQ10 group experienced significantly higher improvement in insulin secretory response than in the control group. There were no side effects during therapy. (Suzuki)

However, other researchers report no observable correlation between serum CoQ10 concentrations and metabolic control in Type I (Eriksson) or Type II (Henriksen) diabetics. They found no significant changes in metabolic parameters during CoQ10 supplementation but reported it did not interfere with glycemic control, and therefore CoQ10 may be used as adjunctive therapy in patients with associated cardiovascular diseases because of the benefits it would provide.

Suggested daily dosage for diabetics: 300 mg. regular CoQ10 or 120 mg. Q-Gel®, the hydrosoluble form.

Herbs and other Beneficial Supplements

Certain herbs hold tremendous therapeutic potential in the regulation of blood sugar levels, and some may also help to prevent some of the complications for which diabetics are at an increased risk.

Gymnema Sylvestre

Gymnema Sylvestre may trigger the regeneration of insulin-producing pancreatic beta cells. Gymnema is an Indian herb which acts a tonifer, or regulator, and it is fairly safe. When drops of gymnema extract are put on the tongue, components in the herb block the sensation of sweetness. People say that taking the herb this way is helpful for stopping sugar cravings.

The extract also boosts production of insulin in people with diabetes, an action that may reduce blood sugar levels and the need for supplemental insulin. In one study, 22 people with Type II diabetes were given gymnema extract along with their regular medications. All had improved blood sugar control, and 21 were able to considerably reduce their dosages of medications. In fact, five of the people were able to discontinue their medications and maintain blood sugar control with the herb alone.

For both Type I and Type II diabetes, the suggested intake for gymnema extract is 400 mg. a day, taken in three or four divided doses. The herb has no apparent side effects. It does not cause low blood sugar and does not affect people whose blood sugar is normal.

If you are on insulin or other blood sugar–lowering drugs, you may want to advise your doctor that you are taking gymnema.

Momordica Charantia

Momordica charantia (bitter melon) is commonly used in Asia, Africa, and other tropical regions to reduce blood sugar levels and help other health problems (psoriasis, HIV). The blood sugar–lowering action of fresh juice or an extract of bitter melon have been clearly established in several studies. Bitter melon has several compounds with confirmed antidiabetic properties.

At least three different groups of constituents in bitter melon have been reported to have blood sugar lowering or other actions of potential benefit in diabetes mellitus. These include a mixture of steroidal saponins known as charantin, insulin-like peptides (polypeptide-p), and alkaloids. (Raman) It is unclear which of these is most effective, or if all three work together.

The polypeptide-p, a protein extracted from bitter melon, has been tested to show an insulin-like activity. When administered to individuals with diabetes mellitus (both Type I and Type II), it exhibits a blood sugar-lowering effect. The polypeptide-p acts on the pancreas, rejuvenating it and activating the dead insulin producing beta cells present in the islets in the pancreas. It also increases the healthy regeneration of beta cells in the pancreas hence increasing the secretion of insulin from the pancreas. As a result, many people are able to reduce their insulin doses to a bare minimum.

This supplement shows absolutely no side effects. It has only been commercially available since 2000.

Bitter melon is safe for those already taking other hypoglycemic drugs or medicine. It is even safe enough for children to use, or as a preventative for nondiabetics, unless you have hypoglycemia (low blood sugar).

Bitter melon also has other health benefits: It reduces cholesterol and triglycerides, helps regulate high blood pressure, and helps reduce nerve damage caused by diabetes leading to numbness and pain in hands, feet and legs.

A small melon can be eaten as food or up to 50 ml. of fresh juice can be drunk per day. For those who do not care for the bitter taste are bitter melon tinctures, of which 5 ml. is generally taken two to three times per day.

Excessively high doses of bitter melon juice can cause abdominal pain and diarrhea. Diabetics taking hypoglycemic drugs (such as chlorpropamide, glyburide, or phenformin) or insulin should use bitter melon under medical supervision, as it may increase the effectiveness of the drugs and lead to severe hypoglycemia.

Momordica extract is also available. For stabilization of blood sugar, the recommended daily dosage is 50 mg.

Other Important Herbs:

- **Fenugreek** may assist insulin in lowering blood sugar levels. Pre-clinical and clinical studies have documented the efficacy of the fiber-rich fraction of fenugreek seeds in the management of diabetes. In Type I and II diabetics, administration of de-fatted, fiber-rich seed significantly reduces fasting blood glucose levels and improves performance in the glucose tolerance test. Fenugreek is also known to help regulate cholesterol.

Researchers have used 5-100 grams daily (one-fifth to three ounces) of de-fatted fenugreek seed powder to control blood sugar swings in diabetes in the short term.

- **Bilberry,** a source of antioxidant anthocyanidins, strengthens capillaries and is used widely in Europe to treat diabetic retinopathy. It also may reduce blood sugar levels.

- **Ginseng,** an adaptogen, lowers blood sugar, and provides physical and mental enhancements in some patients.

- **Ginkgo** strengthens circulatory and nervous system tissues, leading to improved peripheral blood circulation and less chance of vascular damage.

Diabetics frequently develop circulatory problems, especially in the legs. If these problems aren't resolved, the toes, feet, and legs can be damaged by impaired circulation. In worst cases, the damage can lead to amputation. One of the most common reasons for toe, foot, or leg amputations, in fact, is impaired circulation from uncontrolled diabetes.

Ginkgo helps to improve circulation, especially in the smaller arteries in the legs, hands, nerves and brains. It also helps stabilize cell membranes, acts as a powerful antioxidant, and enhances use of oxygen and blood sugar.

The recommend intake of ginkgo for diabetics is 40 mg. three times a day. Look for a standardized extract that contains 24% ginkgoflavoglycosides.

Some people report increased headaches when supplementing ginkgo. If this occurs, discontinue use.

• **5-HTP** (5-Hydroxytryptophan) is a natural derivative of the African-native plant griffonia simplicifonia. As a botanical dietary supplement, no prescription is needed for 5-HTP.

5-HTP acts as a natural anti-depressant. Depression results, in part, from the lack of serotonin, a brain neurotransmitter. Low levels of serotonin are also associated with depression, sleep problems, low threshold for pain, anxiety, overeating, carbohydrate cravings and addictions. Carbohydrate cravings and overeating are commonly associated as predecessors to Type 2 diabetes.

The amino acid L-tryptophan (the precursor to 5-HTP) was used by millions around the world prior to the 1990 to increase 5-hydroxytryptamine (also known as serotonin) levels before it was banned. 5-HTP increases the production of serotonin 10 times more effectively than L-tryptophan.

Many antidepressants prescribed today are selective serotonin reuptake inhibitors (SSRIs). By blocking the reuptake of serotonin, they increase the serotonin available to stimulate serotonin receptors. These include Prozac®, Zoloft®, Paxil®, and Effexor®. While they may be very effective for the treatment of depression, they are not without side effects, including the loss of sex drive. They are also expensive and only available by prescription If you are currently using SSRIs, you may need to reduce your dosage or start at a lower 5-HTP dosage.

Beta endorphins, the "feel-good" hormones, are also significantly elevated after consumption of 200 mg. of 5-HTP by patients with severe depression.

Weight loss products such as Redux and Fenfluramine of the now-banned Phen-Fen diet work by serotonin reuptake inhibition to increase serotonin levels. Beta endorphins seem to fool people into feeling fuller, therefore, individuals eat less and lose weight. Thankfully, 5-HTP does not have any dangerous side effects.

Elevated serotonin levels are associated with:

- Improved sleep
- Decreased depression
- Relief from anxiety
- Weight loss/ suppressed appetite
- Reduced cravings for carbohydrates
- Reduced cravings for alcohol. Alcoholics have depressed levels of serotonin.

For more information on this subject, I recommend reading the book, *Nature's Road to Recovery: Nutritional Supplements for the Alcoholic and Chemical Dependent.*

Other Important Supplements:

Colostrum and IGF-1: Colostrum (also known as "first milk") is rich in numerous immune-enhancing factors which are of great interest to diabetics. Colostrum was not only a first food developed by our Creator, it was our first medicine!

One immune-enhancing factor it contains is Insulin-like Growth Factor-1 (IGF-1). Studies show that plasma levels of IGF-1 in diabetics are lower than those of nondiabetics. IGF-1 stimulates glucose utilization in nondiabetics and seems to benefit diabetics as well. (Dohm)

Depressed IGF-1 levels are associated with many of the complications of diabetes, especially in Type II (Cortizo), such as kidney problems (Segev), weight gain and obesity (Bereket), diabetic retinopathy (Lacka), injury and delayed wound healing (Brown), and possibly vascular complications and cardiovascular disease. (Goke, Bereket)

Researchers at the University of Miami School of Medicine, Florida, have shown that IGF-1 decreases collagen degradation and, therefore, supplemental IGF-1 may have beneficial implications for diabetic complications. (Lupia)

Researchers show that addition of IGF-I supplementation to insulin in adolescents with IDDM can restore circulating IGF-1 levels and thus suppress growth hormone levels and improve insulin sensitivity and glycemic control and decrease insulin requirements. (Dunger)

Bovine Colostrum Increases IGF-1

Several studies show that bovine colostrum supplementation increases serum IGF-1. (Mero, Wester)

Diabetics using colostrum in the form of a lozenge (for sublingual delivery) report lower fasting glucose levels and a reduction in insulin usage. They also report a reduced frequency in infection. Other diabetics using colostrum lozenges report:

- Within 3 days, fasting blood sugar levels upon awakening are normal.
- Within 7 days, insulin use is reduced by one-half.
- Within 30 days, their fingernails have hardened.

Lactoferrin Improves Diabetics' Resistance to Infection and Tissue Damage

Another important protective immune-enhancing component of colostrum is lactoferrin. Lactoferrin is an important enzyme naturally produced in the oral cavity, saliva and tears.

Supplemental lactoferrin may help prevent diabetic infections as it specifically binds to glucose-modified damaged proteins which are elevated among diabetics. Exposure to these damaged proteins is undesirable as the bacterial killing activities of lactoferrin is blocked and the bactericidal and enzymatic activity of lysozyme is inhibited. (Li) Supplementing lactoferrin increases its protective and healing ability throughout the body.

Periodontal Disease

A higher prevalence and severity of periodontal disease is seen in diabetics. Levels of saliva, which contains lactoferrin and other protective components, are significantly lower in IDDM compared to NIDDM or controls. (Ben-Aryeh) Topical applications of lactoferrin products may be beneficial for this reason.

Essential Fatty Acids and Fats

Essential fatty acids (EFAs) are very helpful for diabetics. These are the Omega-6 and the Omega-3s (LNA), made up of EPA (eicosapentaenoic acid) and DHA (docosahexaenoic acid). Omega-3 deficiencies are **very** common, and much more common than Omega-6 deficiencies. Omega-3's can be obtained by regularly eating fatty fish such as salmon, cod, tuna steak, trout, haddock, mackerel and flax seeds. There are no other good food sources. Supplements are available from fish oils, flax seed oil or perilla oil.

Omega-6 fatty acids such as GLA (gamma linoleic acid) protect against the development of diabetic neuropathy, the nerve dysfunction that can result from diabetes. Omega-3s help prevent damage to blood vessels and enhance insulin secretion and help regulate cholesterol and triglyceride levels.

In one study, diabetics who had mild neuropathy demonstrating some nerve damage took 480 mg. a day of GLA for one year. Nerve health was assessed with tests that measured how fast their nerves conducted signals, their muscle strength, and other factors. At the end of the year, all of the functions had improved in the people taking GLA, and most showed significant change for the better.

Diabetics Have Depressed Levels of EFAs

Diabetics commonly have depressed levels of EFAs, especially the Omega-3 fatty acids. Omega-3s improve the body's ability to respond to insulin. They are needed for the healthy structure of the cellular membranes and therefore, a normal response to insulin. Too much Omega-6 (from vegetable oils) actually diminishes the cellular response to insulin.

The high level of glucose in diabetics interferes with their ability to convert LNA into DHA. This is significant for a number of reasons:

1. DHA (and EPA) improve the function of insulin receptors, which helps lower glucose levels.

2. DHA helps lower glucose levels as it increases blood insulin concentrations. (Hamazaki)

3. DHA is an important structural component of the retina. Degeneration of the retina is a common cause of blindness in diabetics.

4. DHA helps regulate blood lipid levels, a risk factor for the development of atherosclerosis. Over 26 published trials have demonstrated the benefits of adding fish oils EPA and DHA to lower triglyceride levels among diabetics, both insulin-dependent (IDDM) and non-insulin dependent (NIDDM). (Friedberg) *Note: Studies were conducted on a dosage level of one gram DHA and one gram EPA per day.*

EFAs Benefit Lipid Levels in Type II Diabetics

Elevated triglycerides, VLDL, and HDL are among the common problems among diabetics increasing the risk of cardiovascular complications. Japanese researchers investigated the effects of EPA and DHA on 21 NIDDM patients. The patients were treated for 28 days with 1.7 grams EPA and 1.15 grams DHA per day. After the DHA/EPA treatment there was a strong decrease in triglycerides and VLDL serum levels, accompanied by a significant increase in HDL. (Haban)

Fish oil studies have also demonstrated that it lowers triglyceride levels effectively by almost 30% and that it has no adverse affects on glucose in diabetics. (Friedberg)

EPA/DHA Increase Glucose Disposal

To determine the impact of fish-oil supplementation on glucose and lipid metabolism in patients with impaired glucose tolerance, eight obese subjects with impaired glucose tolerance (average age 50.3) were given 3.8 grams EPA and 2.5 grams DHA in addition to their regular diet for two weeks. Glucose disposal rate increased after fish-oil supplementation, whereas no change was seen without fish oil. (Fasching)

EFAs and Neuropathy

Neuropathy (painful swelling and destruction of the nerve and nerve endings) is a common problem that accompanies diabetes. Individuals feel numbness, pain and "pins and needles" sensations in their hands and feet with this type of nerve damage. It can make simple tasks like putting on socks or walking down stairs extremely difficult.

Neuropathy can also be the result of drug poisoning (common among individuals taking various medications), lead poisoning and alcoholism. Other causes of neuropathies include viral infection and autoimmune disorders such as arthritis, lupus, and periarteritis (a disease of the small arteries that can lead to hypertension, heart attack, muscle weakness, skin ulcerations, and gangrene, which can lead to amputation). These conditions are accompanied by elevated levels of free radicals and depressed levels of antioxidants.

Experts in the field of fatty acid research, such as Dr. David Horrobin, suspect that this impairment of conversion of LNA to GLA could lead to defective nerve function because metabolites of GLA are known to be important in nerve membrane structure, nerve blood flow, and nerve conduction. GLA supplementation helps correct the impaired nerve function in animal models of diabetes. (Horrobin, Diabetes, 1997)

Supplementation of a combination of GLA, EPA and DHA, plus antioxidant protection through alpha lipoic acid (300 mg. twice daily) can help correct symptoms of diabetic neuropathy. (Cameron, Horrobin)

Sources of EFAs

Omega-6 fatty acids (GLA) are found in borage oil, evening primrose oil or black currant oil. Suggested intake is 500 mg. daily.

Omega-3's are provided by fresh fatty fish such as mackerel, salmon, tuna steak, trout, haddock and freshly ground flax seeds. Fish-oil capsules or supplements of flaxseed or perilla oil are also available. Recommended supplemental intake is 2,000 – 4,000 mg. a day of Omega-3 (EPA/DHA).

Note: Canned fish are not a good source of EFAs as the high temperatures used in canning destroy almost all the essential fatty acids.

Trans-Fatty Acid Dangers

Fats known as trans fatty acids, commonly found in many processed foods (packaged foods like bread, crackers, cookies and other baked goods, chips and other snacks, fried foods including french fries, margarine and all foods containing hydrogenated or partially hydrogenated oils), already have been linked to heart disease and high cholesterol. A study from the Harvard School of Public Health also suggests that limiting their consumption also can greatly lower diabetes risk. (Salmeron)

Consumption of healthy polyunsaturated fats, such as Omega-3 (found in fatty fish and flax) and Omega-6 fatty acids (found in many liquid vegetable oils), is protective against diabetes. Researchers suggest that replacing trans-fats in the diet with polyunsaturated fats can reduce the risk of diabetes by as much as 40%.

Studies now show a link between trans--fatty acid consumption and Type II diabetes. Researchers believe the dramatic increase in consumption of trans-fatty acids (from commercially packaged foods) directly relates to the increase in Type II diabetes. (Hu)

Trans fats are formed when liquid fats are hydrogenated, or partially hydrogenated, to make them solid at room temperature. They are routinely used in commercially sold crackers, baked goods, cereals, and breads because they increase the shelf life of the products. Most restaurants also deep-fry foods in oils containing these trans-fats.

The average American eats approximately five grams of trans-fatty acids per day. That translates into about 7.4% of total daily fat consumed.

Researchers at Harvard found that total fat intake

compared with calories from carbohydrates was not associated with diabetes incidence. They also found no significant link between diabetes and the intake of saturated fats (from animal and dairy products) or between diabetes and monounsaturated fats, from olive, canola and peanut oils. But a significant increase in diabetes risk was associated with consumption of trans-fats. (Hu)

While saturated animal fats have been perceived as the most dangerous fats, the (fake) hardened vegetable oils now appear to be **more dangerous** than saturated fats.

What Foods Contain Trans-Fatty Acids?

Currently, trans-fats are not listed on nutrition labels. To determine which foods contain them, look for hydrogenated oil or partially hydrogenated oil in the ingredients list of processed baked goods. Also stay away from deep-fried foods like french fries when eating out.

By reading food labels and becoming aware of the types of foods containing these fats you can **avoid** trans-fats. Baking and cooking at home where you can control the type of fat you use will also help a great deal.

Avoiding unhealthy processed fat **does not** give you license to consume unlimited amounts of natural fats even though they are from healthier sources such as olive oil or soybean oil.

Trans and Cis Forms

A trans-fatty acid is created when the natural, smooth-shaped "cis" molecule is replaced by a sharp, twisted "trans" molecule. This occurs through hydrogenation which converts fats that are naturally fluid at room temperature to a more solid form, like most animal

48

Fatty Acid Content of Processed Foods

S= saturated fat
MU=monounsaturated fat
PU= polyunsaturated fat
Trans = trans-fatty acids

*Amounts given are **mg. per 100 mg.** consumed*
Random sample brands selected

S	MU	PU	Trans	S	MU	PU	Trans
French-fried potatoes (fast food restaurants-2 selected)				**Popcorn**, oil-popped			
3.8	9.33	1.38	**4.96**	8.18	23.9	3.01	**12.37**
4.64	9.97	1.44	**5.22**				
				Popcorn, microwave-popped			
French-fried potatoes (frozen, unprepared)				5.97	14.99	3.16	**7.65**
1.79	6.22	1.07	**3.38**	**Margarine,** stick			
				9.4	41.92	11.44	**17.31**
Baked biscuits, plain, refrigerated dough				**Margarine,** tub			
2.76	7.54	0.83	**4.06**	12.45	28.83	25.7	**11.29**
				Shortening			
Crackers, cheese, regular				25.43	42.0	27.98	**12.01**
5.94	18.92	3.93	**7.43**	**Shortening**,butter flavor			
Crackers, standard snack-type, regular				24.98	41.63	28.99	**20.84**
3.24	15.01	2.44	**8.18**	**Fats and oils,** spread			
				14.33	41.41	14.37	**22.47**
Cookies, chocolate chip, commercially prepared, regular				**Salad dressing**, ranch			
7.11	15.14	2.66	**9.04**	6.9	15.44	19.1	**3.71**
Cookies, vanilla sandwich with creme filling				**Mayonnaise**			
4.19	13.47	1.18	**7.09**	11.43	22.86	41.91	**3.4**
Cookies, vanilla wafers, reduced fat				**Candy bar,** milk chocolate coated nougat w/ caramel			
2.86	9.43	0.97	**4.25**	9.04	7.43	0.73	**1.6**
Hamburger or hotdog bun, plain				**Candy bar,** milk chocolate coated cookie bar w/caramel			
1.18	2.87	0.96	**1.29**	9.38	13.07	1.33	**6.92**
Tortilla chips				**Frosting,** vanilla, ready-to-eat			
3.57	14.01	6.0	**4.12**	4.37	9.64	2.3	**4.04**

49

fats. This stabilizes the fatty acid, protecting it from rancidity, and makes it an excellent choice (from a commercial standpoint) for products that will be packaged and sit on store shelves indefinitely.

The problem is that the body does not know how to metabolize these man-made fats and they end up causing problems literally from head to toe. Where the body requires the use of fatty acids, such as a structural component for membranes, they just don't work as well as the real thing – and our health suffers for it.

Some researchers strongly believe that these synthetic trans-fatty acids in our food supply are slowly and insidiously wrecking the integrity of our cells. When this synthetic trans-fatty acid gets into cell membrane construction, our cells cannot function optimally. We cannot effectively ward off viruses; the vital biochemical exchanges occurring between the interior and exterior of our cells can be mixed up, and our cellular oxidation is less than nature intended for all our physical and mental needs.

This cellular degeneration is cumulative as we continue to eat these trans-fats. It doesn't improve over time or simply vanish. It slowly gets worse and worse. Because the body was designed to heal itself, if we min-

> *Trans-fatty acids clearly increase diabetes risk. Substituting natural poly-unsaturated fatty acids (EFAs) for trans-fatty acids would likely substantially reduce the risk of Type II diabetes.*

imize our intake, we greatly increase our ability to recover from any damage from previous exposure.

We were told (deceived is a better word) to stop eating butter and to stop cooking with lard and told to eat margarine and vegetable shortening because it was the "healthy thing to do." It's not. It's the opposite.

Scientists, doctors, government and the media have campaigned for the last 40 years to convince us that "saturated" animal fat is harmful and leads to heart disease, cancer, and other degenerative conditions and therefore, margarine, because it contains no cholesterol, is preferable. However, competent scientists have known all along that manufactured fats (margarine and other hydrogenated vegetable oil products) are more harmful than the natural animal fats (such as butter and lard) they replace. Keep in mind, however, that animal fats are saturated fat and we do need to limit our consumption of them as well. Also note that there is no biological need for the body to consume any saturated fats. The liver will produce all the cholesterol the body need and in fact, only produces more with the more cholesterol we consume in our diet. Only the polyunsaturated fats are called "essential," meaning, they cannot be produced in the body and therefore we must obtain them on a daily basis through the diet.

Because animal fats (such as from dairy, eggs, beef, chicken, etc,) are natural and were designed to be used as food, the body is naturally equipped to deal with them in small amounts. It is only in excess that they create problems in the body.

Diet: Making Food Choices

Choosing the correct foods is very important for diabetics. Some physicians believe a diet with 70-80% carbohydrates (such as those recommended by Dean Ornish and Nathan Pritikin) can be helpful. In one study, a diet made up of 70-75% calories from complex carbohydrates, 15-25% protein and 5-10% fats, reduced insulin needs of Type I diabetics by 30-40%.

Others suggest that a very low carbohydrate diet (10-20%) can reduce insulin needs and help maintain stable blood sugars. This requires a severely limited intake of grains, bread, fruits, pasta, and starchy vegetables (potatoes, yams, beans, etc.) and a great increase in fats and protein. While this is a popular weight loss diet, it is very hard on the liver (causes acidosis) and increases cardiac risks long term.

Higher fat diets are higher in saturated fats and cholesterol than current dietary guidelines and their long-term use would increase serum cholesterol levels and risk for coronary heart disease (CHD). While high fat diets may promote short-term weight loss, the potential hazards for worsening risk for progression of atherosclerosis override the short-term benefits. Individuals derive the greatest health benefits from

52

diets low in saturated fat and high in carbohydrate and fiber: these increase sensitivity to insulin and lower risk for CHD. (J.W. Anderson, M.D., Veterans Affairs Medical Center, Internal Medicine, College of Medicine, University of Kentucky, Lexington)

Complex carbohydrates such as found in beans and whole grains are slowly broken down in the body into sugars so that glucose levels do not rise quickly as they do when one eats simple carbohydrates such as in fruit juice or refined carbohydrates such as in sugar or white flour products.

Some practitioners believe that the high incidence of diabetes and the increasing incidence of younger and younger individuals experiencing Type II diabetes is directly related to the typical Western diet of refined, overly-processed foods. It is recommended that individuals follow a diet high in complex carbohydrates and plant fiber.

The latest research demonstrates that eating more fiber-rich cereal and cutting back on sugar can cut the risk of developing diabetes. Although fruits and vegetables supply important nutrients for health, the type of fiber in those foods, according to this study, did not prevent diabetes. The Harvard researchers advise that grains should be consumed in a minimally refined form to reduce the incidence of diabetes. Foods containing rapidly digested carbohydrates such as low-fat sugary desserts, bread or crackers can quickly increase glucose in your blood. This triggers increased insulin levels that may eventually lead to Type II diabetes. Instead, whole grain breads and pasta and unrefined whole grain cereals (like barley and oats) should be eaten.

Our Sugar Habit

Sugar is much like a drug. It has addictive properties and adverse side effects. Sugar is not a whole natural food and does not even resemble the original sources that God made – sugar cane and sugar beets. Sugar is highly refined, fragmented, denatured, and completely stripped of almost all nutrients that were present in its original form. The final processed result is a pure crystallized form of sucrose, a white "pharmaceutically pure" chemical. In contrast, sugar cane and sugar beets are natural and contain minerals, vitamins, trace elements, enzymes, essential fatty acids, amino acids and very important **fiber**.

Eating sugar actually creates **a loss** of essential nutrients (such as B vitamins, chromium, etc.) which are required to metabolize sugar in the body. Interestingly, in the processing of raw sugar cane or sugar beets, **over 90% of the naturally-occurring chromium and other important nutrients are lost.** Chromium is specifically needed for insulin to bring glucose into the cells to be used as fuel (that's why God put it in foods that contain carbohydrates). Without chromium, we can't burn these calories, so instead they are converted to fat and stored away.

Compared to sugar, honey could practically be considered health food because honey contains several minerals and nutrients to assist in the body's use of the carbohydrate, yet the Bible clearly warns us not to eat too much honey (Proverbs 25:27).

In addition to causing weight problems, sugar is a major contributing factor in the development of many degenerative conditions such as diabetes, heart disease, tooth decay, periodontal disease and osteoporosis. Sugar consumption has also been associated with criminal behavior and hyperactivity in children.

Whole foods such as whole grains, beans, vegetables, fruits, etc., are digested slowly and changed into forms of sugar the body can use for energy and for its vital functioning. But refined concentrated sugar is rapidly absorbed into the bloodstream rapidly raising the level of sugar in the blood to a dangerously high level. At this point one will temporarily feel an abundance of energy.

This puts a tremendous burden upon the pancreas. It overreacts, dumping an excess amount of insulin into the bloodstream in order for the elevated sugar level to be normalize. **If** the body has adequate levels of chromium, B vitamins and other nutrients needed to complete this process, and if the energy can be used (unlikely, amongst the sedentary lifestyles so prevalent today), the glucose can enter the cells to be burned.

The excess insulin not only rapidly brings the sugar level down, it lowers it **far below normal**. The term associated with this is **hypoglycemia (low blood sugar).** When this happens, one can experience a number of unpleasant symptoms such as sleepiness, irritability, headaches, anxiety, insomnia, poor memory, weight gain, sweet cravings, depression, crying spells, cold fingers and toes, blurred vision, dry eyes, etc.

A diet high in sugar or simple carbohydrates compounded by stress, overwork, skipping meals, etc., can establish a pattern of rapidly rising, then rapidly falling blood sugar levels, causing fatigue, headaches, irritability, fainting, blurred eyes, mental confusion, memory lapse, light headedness, etc.

Many adults have poor insulin function – diabetic or not! Normal amounts of insulin are produced and released into the bloodstream, but because of the high sugar diet, it is present in the blood more often than not. The cells eventually become less sensitive to this continual presence of insulin. Like the first few times the fire alarm goes off, we jump in response to it, but if it continually keeps ringing, we eventually ignore it.

Elevated insulin levels in the blood stream quickly causes weight gain. In fact, most of our body fat results from consumption of sugar (carbohydrates), not fat! This is driven by the effects of insulin and proven in the insulin-resistant (Type II) diabetic. By control insulin secretion through diet, individuals are able to significantly reduce body fat, cholesterol, diabetes and heart disease. Diet can also regulate secretion of another pancreatic hormone (glucagon), which has additional beneficial effects on fat metabolism and sugar regulation.

Sugar accounts for approximately 24% of our total caloric intake. On average, Americans consume over 30 teaspoons of sugar per day per person. Remember, some people consume much less, so that means some people are taking in **much more** than the average.

We realize that candy, desserts and sweets contain sugar, but do you realize how much? In addition, sugar may be found in many places we would not even dream of looking: salt, peanut butter, bread, fruit juices, instant oatmeal, meat products, canned vegetables, spaghetti sauce, mayonnaise, toothpaste, baby food, etc. Many so-called "healthy" breakfast cereals are actually loaded with sugar.

Because of the bad reputation sugar is getting (and

rightfully so), many manufacturers give sugar other names which we may not immediately identify in label reading. These include: corn syrup, corn syrup solids, maple syrup, molasses, cane syrup, fructose, dextrose, maltose, lactose, etc.

Estimated teaspoons of sugar per serving:

Hard candy (4 oz.) 20
Hostess Iced Honey Cupcake (1 piece) 13
Apple pie (1 slice) 12
Chocolate candy bar (3 Musketeers) 11
Starburst Chews (2.07 oz.) 11
Cola beverage (12 oz.) 10
Sherbet (1/2 cup) 9
Flavored yogurt (8 oz.) 7
Ice cream (4 oz.) 5
Orange marmalade (1 Tbs.) 5
Ketchup (1 Tbs.) 1

Estimated grams of sugar per serving (1/2 – 3/4 cup):

General Mills Honey Nut Cheerios 10
General Mills Wheaties Honey Gold 10
Kellogg's Fruitiful or Raisin Bran 9
General Mills Raisin Nut Bran 8
Kellogg's Branbuds 8

Percentage of refined white table sugar by weight:

Non-dairy creamer 60%
Milk chocolate candy 50%
Chocolate cake 36%
Salad dressings . . . . .up to 30%
Lucky Charms 50%
Cocoa Pebbles 54%
Apple Jacks 55%
Sugar Smacks 61%

Obesity is associated with a greater risk of Type II diabetes. For over 50 years we have known that glucose tolerance can be improved by reducing body weight.

Maintaining normal weight is also the primary factor in diabetes prevention. Avoidance of refined sugars not only helps keep your weight down, but it also very simply may prevent diabetes.

Aspartame

Aspartame, a high intensity, non-caloric sweetener, is used extensively worldwide in over 5,000 products. The high consumption of this dangerous sugar replacement (also called NutraSweet®, Equal®) is just about as disturbing as the high intake of sugar.

I visited several diabetes web sites and when viewing the recipes I was very disappointed to see page after page of recipes for desserts and sweets containing aspartame. We need to be replacing desserts and sweets with nutritious wholesome health-promoting foods.

Aspartame Is TOXIC To The Body!

The best-selling book, *Prescription for Nutritional Healing* by James and Phyllis Balch lists aspartame under the category of "Chemical Poisons."

Upon ingestion, aspartame is metabolized to two amino acids (phenylalanine and aspartic acid) and methanol. (Trefz) Methanol qualifies as an exceptionally toxic substance, even at very low doses. (Roe) The minimum methanol amount needed to cause death (without medical treatment) is 300-1000 mg./kg. This is equivalent to only 0.85 - 2.85 oz. for a 154 lb. (70 kg.) man (much less for a child). (Kavet)

The amount of methanol needed to cause acute toxicity varies widely from person to person (Kavet). The interaction of methanol exposure with exposure to other chemicals or drugs may decrease or increase methanol toxicity. (Posner)

The absorption of methanol into the body speeds up considerably when free methanol is ingested. Free methanol is created from aspartame when it is heated to above 86° Fahrenheit (30° Centigrade). This occurs when aspartame-containing product is improperly stored or when it is cooked or heated (e.g., as part of a "food" product such as sugar-free gelatin or pudding).

In the body, methanol is oxidized to formaldehyde and formic acid, which are both toxic. Formaldehyde is a deadly neurotoxin (*neuro* referring to brain cells). An Environmental Protection Agency (EPA) assessment of methanol states that methanol is considered a cumulative poison due to its low rate of excretion once it is absorbed. They recommend limiting consumption to 7.8 mg./day. A one-liter, aspartame-sweetened beverage contains about 56 mg. of methanol. (Monte)

Symptoms from methanol poisoning include headaches, ear buzzing, dizziness, nausea, gastrointestinal disturbances, weakness, vertigo, chills, memory lapses, numbness and shooting pains in the extremities, behavioral disturbances and neuritis. The most well known problems from methanol poisoning are vision problems (misty vision, contraction of visual fields, blurring, obscuration of vision, retinal damage and blindness). Formaldehye, a known carcinogen, causes retinal damage, interferes with DNA replication, and causes birth defects. (U.S. F.D.A.)

Aspartame accounts for over 75% of the adverse reactions to food additives reported to the U.S. Federal Drug Agency (F.D.A.). These reactions, which include seizures and death, were disclosed in a February 1994 Department of Health and Human Services report. A few of the 90 different documented symptoms listed as being caused by aspartame include: (Kavet, Monte)

Headaches/Migraines	Dizziness
Numbness	Muscle spasms
Weight gain	Rashes
Fatigue	Insomnia
Memory loss	Vision problems
Hearing loss	Heart palpitations
Breathing difficulties	Anxiety attacks
Slurred speech	Tinnitus
Vertigo	Joint pain

Some researchers and physicians studying the adverse effects of aspartame report the following can be triggered or worsened by ingesting aspartame: (Stoddard)

Brain tumors	Multiple sclerosis
Epilepsy	Chronic fatigue syndrome
Parkinson's disease	Alzheimer's
Mental retardation	Lymphoma
Fibromyalgia	Diabetes

One liter of diet pop contains about 56 mg. of methanol – about 7 times the E.P.A. daily limit.

Anytime you see "reduced calorie," "sugar free," or "diet," you need to find out what substance replaces the sugar. Aspartame is often found in the following products: Soft drinks, over-the-counter and prescription drugs (often listed under "inactive ingredients"), vitamin and herb supplements, yogurt, instant breakfasts, candy, sweets and desserts, breath mints, cereals, sugar-free chewing gum, juice beverages, laxatives, milk drinks, shake mixes, tabletop sweeteners, cocoa mixes, coffee and tea beverages, instant teas and coffees, topping mixes, wine coolers, etc.

FOR MORE INFORMATION READ:

Excitotoxins: The Taste That Kills by Russell L. Blaylock, M.D., Health Press, Santa Fe, New Mexico, 1994, ISBN 0-929173-14-7. Dr. Blaylock is an Associate Professor of Neurosurgery at the Medical University of Mississippi.

Aspartame (NutraSweet) - Is it Safe? by H.J. Roberts, MD. Available from the Aspartame Consumer Safety Network.

Stevia: Sugar and Aspartame Alternative

Stevia comes from the dried leaves of the stevia plant originally from the rain forests of Brazil and Paraguay. Today it is also grown in Japan, Korea, Thailand and China. It is an excellent alternative to sugar. It has no calories, has none of the side effects or health risks of sugar, aspartame and saccharin and is not broken down by heat.

The natives in South America used stevia primarily as a sweetener, a practice adopted by European colonists in local regions. The indigenous tribes also used stevia to treat diabetes. (Leung)

The greatest use of stevia today is found in Japan. The Japanese have used stevia for 25 years as a sugar substitute in their manufacture of "American" products like diet Coke and Wrigley's sugarless gum. Stevia accounts for nearly 40% of the sweetener market in Japan. Due to more strict safety restrictions, aspartame and saccharin are banned. Stevia is also commonly used in various parts of South America.

In the United States, stevia is not marketed as a sweetener, but as a dietary supplement due to federal regulations.

Stevia contains glycosides, especially stevioside, which give stevia its sweetness. Stevioside is about 30-50 times sweeter than sugar, but it contains no calories. It can be used in cooking and baking in many cases just as sugar is – you simply use much less. A number of good stevia cookbooks are also available.

Stevia has beneficial effects on glucose tolerance and

Sweeteners Available

Use!	Avoid!
Stevia *	Aspartame (NutraSweet, Equal, Canderel)
Barley malt	Neotame
Evaporated cane juice	Sucralose (Splenda)
Fruit juice	Acesulfame-K (Sunette, Sweet & Safe, Sweet One)
Rice syrup	Cyclamates
Honey	Saccharin
Licorice root ^	Refined sugar
Fructooligosaccharides (FOS)	High fructose sweeteners
Amasake	Sugar alcohols (xylitol, sorbitol)^
Lo Han Kuo Extract (Chinese fruit)	

Safe for diabetics   ^ *Use in small amounts*

is therefore helpful for diabetics. (Curi) A recent study in Denmark showed that stevioside and steviol stimulate insulin secretion via a direct action on beta cells. The results indicate that the compounds indeed have a potential role as antihyperglycemic agents in the treatment of Type II diabetes. (Jeppesen)

Its use as a sweetener could reduce one's intake of sugars, reducing our caloric intake. Usually, the powdered herb is added directly to food or beverages.

Stevia also has other benefits as it promotes probiotic growth in the intestinal tract and reduces hypertension (as recently shown in a human double-blind placebo-controlled study. (Chan) Extensive reviews of human and animal data indicate stevia to be safe. (Blumenthal)

For many recipes, one cup sugar can be replaced with 1 1/2 teaspoons powdered stevia extract.

Apple Pie

Pastry for a 9-inch, 2-crust pie
6 cups peeled and thinly sliced pie apples such as Jonathan or Winesap
1 - 2 tsp. fresh lemon juice
1 1/2 tsp. Stevia Extract Powder
2 - 3 tbsp. whole wheat pastry flour
1/4 tsp. nutmeg
1 tsp. cinnamon
Dash of cloves or allspice
2 tbsp. butter

Fit bottom pastry into a pie dish. In a large mixing bowl sprinkle lemon juice over apples and stir to mix. Using a cup or small bowl stir together stevia, flour, nutmeg, cinnamon, and cloves or allspice. Sprinkle spice mixture over apples and carefully stir to coat apples. Pile apples into bottom crust. Dot with butter.

With water, moisten the outer rim of the lower crust. Place upper crust on pie and crimp edges together. Slit top of pie to allow steam to escape. Place on a cookie sheet. Bake at 350° in a preheated oven for 55 - 60 minutes. Aluminum foil can be placed over the pie during the last 15 minutes to prevent over-browning. Cool on a rack, cover and leave at room temperature overnight or refrigerate if you like.

Fresh Lemonade: Yields about 2 quarts

1 cup fresh lemon juice (from about 5 lemons)
1-2 tsp. Stevia Extract Powder (depends on sweetness desired)
7 cups water

Place the lemon juice, stevia and water in a 2 quart glass jar. Stir briefly to dissolve the stevia. Cover and refrigerate. Adjust the amount of lemon juice and stevia as desired. To serve over ice, reduce the water to 6 cups.

Easy, No-Bake Chocolate Silk Pie
Yields about 6 servings

1 box extra firm tofu
1/2 cup cocoa powder
2 tsp. Stevia Extract Powder
Mix thoroughly in food processor or blender.
Spoon into graham cracker pie crust. Smooth.

Top with fresh whipped topping sweetened with stevia. Garnish with fresh strawberries if desired.

Stevia-Sugar Recipe Conversion

1 cup sugar = 24 packets **OR**
12 tsp. Stevia Blend **OR**
2 1/2 tsp. Stevia Liquid Extract **OR**
1 1/2 tsp. Pure Extract (Stevioside)

Weight Control

Americans seem to ignore their risk of developing diabetes as only 1 in 25 of respondents to a Gallup poll cited diabetes a health concern in those who were 25-35 pounds overweight. Diabetes **should** be a **big** concern as more than 80% of people with adult-onset (Type II diabetes) are significantly overweight.

According to Jerry Franz, Vice President of Communications for the American Diabetes Association:

Adults who are 20-30% overweight are more likely to develop insulin-dependent diabetes, and risk gets higher as weight increases. A weight loss of 10-15 pounds, combined with a treatment regimen of nutrition and exercise can often be effective in keeping blood glucose close to normal.

From a Biblical Perspective

From a Biblical perspective, fasting is strongly encouraged. There are many types of fasting and many reasons to fast, but the health reasons are definitely nothing to be ignored.

Fasting was done during mourning or times of great stress. We often do the opposite – turning to food for comfort during such times – overeating, instead of cutting back. This actually creates even more stress on the body. Everything we eat, the body must go to work on to break it down, use what it needs, and eliminate or store the rest.

Eating for the purposes of simply sustaining the needs of the body is a concept practically abandoned in today's society of abundance. We eat because we feel like it, because it tastes good, because we are bored, or stressed, because it is there. How many times have you started eating something just because a bowl of it was sitting on the table next to you? You may have even thought, "Why am I eating this? I'm not hungry and it doesn't even taste that good!"

Overeating, eating when we are not hungry, eating foods lacking in nutritional value (such as refined foods) creates a great deal of extra work for the body (not to mention added pounds). When we eat like this, the stomach has to continually produce and secrete digestive enzymes and digestive acids, the pancreas has to continually produce insulin, continually taking the components from the body they need to produce these things.

What happens over time? The stomach can no longer produce adequate amounts of hydrochloric acid and now we have a nation addicted to Tums and Malox because we **think** we have indigestion. More often, the problem is not too much acid, it is not enough! If you have digestive problems (discomfort, burping and gas) after eating, the best thing to do is take a few tablespoons of apple cider vinegar with your meals – and eat less! Give your digestive system a break once in a while. Eat more raw foods and chew them thoroughly. Fasting an occasional evening meal is a great help and fasting one day a week is even better. The Bible tells us that the Jews and Gentiles fasted two days a week.

If your blood sugar levels are too low (or unstable) to fast completely, you could do a partial fast such as eating only vegetables (preferably raw). A fast containing only fruits and vegetables is often referred to as a Daniel Fast. (Daniel 1:8-17)

According to Roy Walford, researcher and author of *The 120-Year Diet*, we could plan on living 30 to 50 years longer than we originally expected if we consumed less calories – a lot less calories.

A number of studies have shown that the life span of animals can be extended by restricting their food intake. Rats fed 40% fewer calories lived 50% longer than their unrestricted peers. That corresponds to humans living to be 150 -160 years old.

Walford and a number of others have shown that cutting calories in young animals delays a loss of heart muscle function that ordinarily occurs with aging and can extend the reproductive years. Fewer calories keep their immune systems from deteriorating with age.

A calorically restricted (average of 1,780 calories /day), low-fat (10% of calories), nutrient-dense diet in humans has a large number of health benefits. Such a diet significantly lowers weight in men and women, lowers blood glucose, lowers total leukocyte count, reduces cholesterol levels and decreases blood pressure. (Walford)

Enhanced Use of Insulin

Reducing calories by 52% can extend maximum life span by approximately 33% and increase insulin receptors 15% to 25%. Increased insulin receptors allow us to more efficiently use the energy from the food we eat. Thus, reducing total calorie intake also enhances nutrient intake.

Free Radical Protection

Oxidation is part of the natural metabolic process of the body. Less food eaten means less oxidation and fewer free radicals produced. (Simic) Reducing calories may retard aging based on the reduced production of mitochondrial free radicals. (Feuers) The less food we consume, the less work it is for the body to process and metabolize it.

Reduce Risk Factors for Heart Disease

Improving fatty acid composition of serum lipids benefits Type II diabetics. Individuals undergoing dietary therapy had greater weight loss, better metabolic control and greater improvement in blood lipids than controls.

Researchers have found that dietary strategies are highly effective in reducing other risk factors associated with cardiovascular diseases. To study the role of diet in cardiovascular-risk-factor intervention, 458 high-risk individuals were asked to eat a cardiovaso-protective diet. Such a diet is high in complex carbohydrates, vegetable protein, fiber, vitamin C, potassium and magnesium. Fats consumed consisted largely of polyunsaturated fats, avoiding saturated fat and cholesterol. Fat intake should be about 20% of the total caloric intake. After one year, there was a significant decrease in total risk factors:

- **Significant reduction in blood cholesterol and blood lipid profile**
- **Reduced blood pressure**
- **Reduced weight**

Fiber

Fiber is a carbohydrate food component that is not digested and broken down as are other carbohydrates, or proteins and fats. Fiber (such as cellulose, lignin and pectins) passes through the stomach to the small and large intestine virtually unchanged.

Fiber contains no calories. It provides us with no energy or nutritional value. Its value lies in what the fiber does while it is in the body.

Dietary patterns have changed dramatically over the last century. Modernization and processing continue to increase the distance between a natural food and the food on the table. Removal of fiber plays a great part.

The more a food is processed, the more profitable it is for the manufacturer: Did you know that baking potatoes may cost 35-45 cents a pound, but a pound of potato chips costs about $4.20?

Many common health problems are linked to our lack of fiber intake. Denis Burkitt, M.D., the man who achieved fame for identifying and curing the first human cancer caused by a virus (known as Burkitt's Lymphoma), studied American and African dietary patterns and the differences in health problems. He concluded that lack of fiber was the critical factor, followed by use of refined sugar and white flour. Hippocrates actually used whole grains as medical treatments. Wherever Westernization of dietary habits travels, disease follows. Obesity is first seen, followed by diabetes, appendicitis, gallstones, heart disease and so on. Constipation would be nonexistent if we would eat foods in their natural states without processing.

Centuries ago the refining of grains began. Now, cereal fiber is a rarity instead of the norm. If you want to purchase real whole grain cereals such as millet, rye, buckwheat, wheat, flax or amaranth, you usually have to go to a health food store. Most whole wheat breads are soft, airy white breads with a little wheat bran added for color. Real whole grain bread is very dense, weighing three or four times more than soft white bread.

Effect of Fiber on Insulin

Removing fiber from a naturally high carbohydrate food, dumps too much sugar into your bloodstream, causing production of too much insulin. The job of insulin is to "take" the glucose into the cells to be burned for energy. Too much insulin initiates an enzyme to tell our brain that there is too much glucose, and any excess will be stored.

Removing fiber (for example, when you squeeze an orange to produce orange juice), allows the carbohydrates to rapidly convert into simple sugars and to quickly enter the bloodstream. The pancreas releases a larger amount of insulin to compensate. Insulin triggers the enzyme to tell the body to start storing the excess glucose.

To maintain stable blood sugar and insulin levels, it is far better to eat the whole orange, than to drink the juice and throw away the fiber. In addition, notice how much more satisfied and full you feel after eating a whole apple (which also has less calories) compared to drinking a glass of apple juice.

Benefits of a High Fiber Diet

The health benefits of a high-fiber diet are too numerous to list. Fiber is simply a necessary dietary component that really went unnoticed until we started suffering the effects of eating a diet without it.

Different fiber sources have different effects on the intestinal tract. The effects of soluble fiber, such as psyllium husks, are different than the effects of insoluble fiber such as wheat bran. Both types are important and necessary for good health. Both types of fiber help provide a feeling of fullness and satisfaction to our appetite.

As fiber travels through the digestive tract it takes with it fatty debris from the intestinal tract that would otherwise contribute to weight gain and formation of excess gasses.

In the colon, fiber holds onto water, which helps form a softer, larger, more consistent bowel movement. Fiber also carries bile and excess fats out of the body. Without fiber, much of this fat is reabsorbed and recirculated through the body, and is likely to be stored.

By helping cleanse fat and debris from the digestive tract, nitrogen and sulphur gasses are also reduced, allowing for more optimal absorption of important nutrients, including oxygen, which increases the metabolic rate in the body and is important for memory and energy levels.

One fiber study for the treatment of obesity and elevated cholesterol levels demonstrated how just the daily addition of 15 grams (2 tsp.s) of a high-fiber food supplement could result in a significant weight loss and also a drop in blood cholesterol levels. (Kaul)

Fiber Benefits

- Fiber helps you feel full and eat less.

- Fiber lowers blood sugar and blood pressure.

- Fiber holds water and increases fecal bulk.

- Fiber binds bile acids carrying them (and fats) out of the body.

- Fiber reduces or normalizes transit time. (The time it takes for the food to travel from the mouth to the elimination channels.) This helps reduce toxin levels in the body.

- Fiber causes fermentation in the large bowel (it provides something for the friendly bacteria to grow upon). This aids digestion and helps to keep candida yeast levels in check.

- Fiber is a natural laxative. It helps fight constipation and bloating and improves colon health by "keeping things moving."

- Fiber helps eliminate toxins and waste products faster.

- Fiber lowers the risk of colon-rectal cancer – the second leading cause of death in the U.S.

- Fiber reduces elevated cholesterol.

- Fiber lowers the risk of heart disease – the leading cause of death in the U.S.

- Fiber is a natural, inexpensive approach to health and longevity.

Fiber Content in Foods

<u>Highest to Lowest</u>

1. **Whole grain cereals:** whole grain wheat, rice, corn, barley, rye, buckwheat, millet, oats, amaranth and flax

2. **Legumes:** peas, beans, lentils, **nuts, seeds, and dried fruits**

3. **Root vegetables:** potatoes, yams, kohlrabi, carrots, parsnips, turnips, beets

4. **Fruits** and **leafy vegetables:** lettuce, cabbage, celery, broccoli, cauliflower, etc.

5. **Animal products** contain **no fiber:** Beef, pork, chicken, fish and other meats, eggs, milk and milk products such as cheese, yogurt, etc.

Whole Foods

Nature has a plan for everything. The whole basis behind nature is for everything to work together – nothing in isolation – to use everything to its full potential, wasting nothing.

A more natural diet satisfies hunger because it satisfies the body's real hunger for nutrition. Processing removes components of a food that the body needs to use that particular food to its fullest extent. There are many examples we can use to further demonstrate:

- Fruits and vegetables should not be peeled because the peelings contain vitamins, trace minerals, bioflavonoids and many other important trace components, many of which may not even be identified yet. Buy organic to avoid pesticide residue.

- Most fruits (and many vegetables) are high in sugar (mostly fructose), but the fiber they contain slows down its absorption into the bloodstream preventing too much insulin from being released. It is far better to eat a raw, whole piece of fruit than to just drink the juice and throw away the fiber.

Flax Seed

Flax seed is an excellent whole food high in fiber. It is rich in very important nutritional components which are otherwise hard to find: lignins, a cancer-fighting fiber and also the Omega 3 essential fatty acids (linolenic). Flax seed contains approximately 60% linolenic acid (LNA), and is probably the best source of Omega 3. It also contains the other essential fatty acids, 16% Linoleic (Omega 6), and 18% Oleic (Omega 9).

Flax seeds are also an excellent source of soluble lignin fiber. Flax seed lignins have a very solid amount of research demonstrating their anti-cancer effects, specifically uterine, cervical and breast cancer. Other research has demonstrated the ability of flax seed lignins to reduce blood lipids by as much as 27%. (Cunnane)

Other nutrients provided by flax seed include vitamin E, beta carotene, calcium, magnesium, manganese, potassium and high-quality protein.

What to do with freshly-ground flax seeds:

- Mix with nonfat yogurt, cottage cheese, cheese dips, etc. (the fiber helps the body rid itself of fat, especially saturated fats found in dairy products).

- Mix about 1/4 cup into meat loaf, meat or soy balls.

- Mix about 1/3 cup into homemade breads, waffles, pancakes, muffins or other baked goods.

- Sprinkle 1-2 Tbsp. (per serving) onto salads, scrambled eggs, breakfast cereal (hot or cold), rice or steamed vegetables.

- Blend into protein or fruit shakes or even juice (about 2 Tbsp. per serving). See pg. 78 for sample recipe.

Do not add flax at the stove to things like soup or cooked cereal, add it at the table instead. The fatty acids in flax seed are highly susceptible to destruction and rancidity by exposure to heat, light and oxygen. This is why it is important to use flax freshly ground. Try to prepare an amount which can be consumed right away and refrigerate or freeze any unused portions and use as soon as possible (within 1-2 days).

Oats
An Excellent Food Choice for Glucose Regulation!

A Harvard study reported that eating oatmeal on a regular basis can reduce the risk for Type II diabetes (and therefore also serve as a treatment). The 10-year study followed the diets of over 75,000 American women. They discovered that women who consumed higher levels of oatmeal had the lowest rates of Type II diabetes. The results showed that eating one serving (one cup cooked) oats 2-4 times per week was linked to 16% reduced risk. one serving 5-6 times per week was linked to a 39% risk reduction! (Liu)

Beta glucan is the phytochemical responsible for many of the health-promoting, glucose-regulating, cholesterol-lowering and immune-enhancing effects of oats. Beta glucan is also found in barley, several species of medicinal mushrooms and it is available as a nutritional supplement. Significant quantities (three grams) must be taken to have a beneficial effect on glucose and cholesterol levels. Lower quantities (500-1,000 mg.) are needed to obtain it's immune stimulating effects.

Glycemic response was studied in children with insulin-dependent diabetes at Barbara Davis Center for Childhood Diabetes, Department of Pediatrics, University of Colorado Health Sciences Center, Denver. They found that the most effective "meal" (providing a slow increase and decline in blood sugar levels) contained complex carbohydrates, protein and some fat (such as found in oats). Addition of protein and fat clearly delays the glycemic response. (Wang)

Oatmeal-Flax Muffins

1 1/2 cups old-fashioned oats
1 1/2 cups fat-free buttermilk
Combine and let soak together about 15 minutes.
Add:
1/3 cup brown sugar <u>or</u> 1/4 cup honey
2-3 Tbs. applesauce (optional)
2 eggs or 3 egg whites
1/4 cup freshly-ground flax seed (in coffee bean
      grinder or regular blender)
1 cup whole wheat flour (approximate)
1/2 tsp. baking soda
1 1/2 tsp. baking powder
1/2 tsp. salt

Options to add:
Cinnamon (1 tsp.)
Cardamon (1/2 tsp.) and a pinch of cloves
Raisins
Chopped apple
Grated orange peel and 2 tsp. of frozen orange juice
      concentrate and dried cranberries

Pour into and bake in muffin tins in 400° oven
for 20 minutes. Yield: about 12.

Soy Protein
Improves Blood Lipids /Protects the Heart

Because of the high risk of heart disease for diabetics and the evidence that soy protein improves blood lipid profiles, researchers in Denmark wanted to investigate the potential benefits of soy for diabetics.

In a double-blind crossover trial they found that a high-isoflavone soy protein supplement (50 grams daily) in Type II diabetics resulted in significantly lower LDL cholesterol. Total cholesterol, triglycerides, and homocysteine levels also improved. No change occurred in HDL cholesterol or glucose. The results indicate beneficial effects of dietary soy supplementation on cardiovascular risk markers in Type II diabetics. This improvement is seen even in individuals with near-normal lipid values. (Hermanson)

Fruti Tofu Smoothie
Place in blender:

1/2 cup frozen raspberries or strawberries

1/2 cup cranberries or chopped apple

1/2 cup cranberry (or other similar) juice

2 Tbs. freshly-ground flax seeds

1/3 cup (about 1/2 box) lite tofu

Blend and enjoy!

Yield: 1-2 servings

For a thinner smoothie, add more juice or sparkling mineral water.

Any fresh or frozen fruit can be substituted.

Soy protein powder can be substituted for tofu. Tofu is a cultured soybean product found in the produce or health food section in most markets.

Foods To Help Regulate Glucose (and Hunger)

The goal is to maintain stable glucose levels. Recent recommendations for the dietary management of diabetes mellitus state that diet needs to be individualized so that there is improved glucose and lipid control in the patient. In a majority of individuals with diabetes, this is best done with a diet that is low in fat and high in complex carbohydrates, particularly those of cereal origin.

The best cereal products for this purpose are **barley** and **oats** which are particularly high in the soluble fiber beta glucan. When taken with a meal, beta glucan slows down absorption of carbohydrates in the small intestine. A 50% reduction in glycemic peak can be achieved with a concentration of 10% beta glucan in a cereal food.

A significant lowering of plasma LDL cholesterol concentrations can also be anticipated with the daily consumption of at least three grams of beta glucan. (Wursch, Pick)

You can control your blood sugar levels by the food

Diabetics can benefit from diets high in beta-glucan, as found in oats and barley.

choices and food combinations you make.

- Avoid refined foods (sugar, white flour, sweets, chips, crackers, ready-to-eat cereals)

- Eat whole natural foods the way God made them; minimize cooking whenever possible.

- Barley can be added to soups or casseroles instead of pasta noodles which have a much higher glycemic index. Barley (cooked in chicken or beef broth) also makes an excellent and tasty side dish.

- Oats make an excellent breakfast choice or oat meal (and also ground flax seeds) can be added to baked goods, pancakes, muffins, etc. to lower the glycemic index.

- Eat healthy food combinations by eating a carbohydrate food with a protein or fat.

For example, eating a piece of cheese on your cracker or adding cream cheese or unsweetened peanut butter to your bagel will greatly slow down the glucose response compared to eating the carbohydrate food alone. If you are sensitive to eating fruit (such as bananas, grapes or melon), eat some unsweetened plain yogurt along with it.

When the blood sugar is low the brain produces neurotransmitters to tell you that you are hungry. Your brain decides what to eat. Each food we eat affects us in a different way. Some foods are more satisfying to our hunger than others. An apple may be more satisfying than a chocolate chip cookie, even though they have approximately the same number of calories. Sometimes you can eat something, feel satisfied and then be hungry again in 10 minutes when your blood sugar quickly falls as fast as it rose (from eating a refined carbohydrates).

When you eat, as your blood sugar rises, insulin is released telling the cells to start burning off the glucose. Some foods cause the blood sugar level to increase more quickly and to a higher level than others. A dramatic rise in blood sugar corresponds to a dramatic rise in insulin and a rapid fall of glucose.

Low (and steady) insulin levels:

- Promote calorie and fat burning.

- Help minimize hunger and food cravings.

Elevated (spiked) insulin levels:

- Stimulate the appetite.

- Cause blood sugar to fall rapidly and to very low levels causing fatigue, irritability and more hunger.

- Cause fewer calories to be burned and more to be stored as fat. Note: Elevated triglyceride levels usually come from stored excess sugars!

Glycemic Index

The glycemic index is a rating system indicating how different foods affect the rise in blood sugar. Foods that have the most dramatic affect on blood sugar are rated higher. Table sugar, which is rated 100, has the most dramatic effect on blood sugar levels, and therefore, receives the highest score.

Eat more low glycemic index foods that promote a slow, moderate rise in blood sugar and insulin after eating them. This helps keep hunger in check and encourage the body to dissolve body fat by converting it into energy. These foods allow you to consume more calories without gaining weight. They actually increase your metabolic rate.

Avoid high glycemic index foods. These cause sudden, unstable swings in blood sugar, first with rapid, very high sugar and insulin surges, followed by a crash of sugar to excessively low levels. These foods increase your cravings for simple carbohydrates, sweets, etc., causing overeating and bingeing.

- Increase foods high in soluble fiber such as lentils and beans, which have a lower glycemic response.

- Fat lowers a glycemic rating of a food because it slows absorption of the sugars. Even though they are high in sugar, regular ice cream and yogurt, have a lower glycemic rate because of their high fat content. Reduced fat and non-fat varieties have much higher glycemic index rates.

- Juiced and pureed fruits and vegetables have a higher glycemic rating than the whole fruit or vegetable.

- Generally, the longer you cook foods that are primarily carbohydrates (like potatoes or vegetables), the more simple the sugars become and the higher the glycemic rating.

- The more you alter a food (through processing), the higher the glycemic index rating becomes. Mashed potatoes have a higher rate than whole potatoes. Rice flour has a higher rate than whole rice. The more intact (natural) the food is, the healthier your insulin response will be after eating it. Coarsely-ground flour has a lower index rating than finely ground flour.

High Glycemic Index Foods

AVOID these foods to minimize insulin increases!

GLYCEMIC INDEX

Sugar, corn syrup	100
Dates	100
Hard liquor	95
Rice (instant)	91
Carrot juice	90
Puffed rice cereal	90
Rice Chex cereal	89
Honey	87
Cakes and most desserts	70-87
Corn flakes cereal	84
Potatoes (baked)	84
Potatoes (instant)	84
Pretzels	83
Rice Krispies cereal	82
Rice cakes	82
Dried figs	80
Jelly beans	80
Angel food cake	77
Vanilla wafers	77
Potato chips, corn chips	60-77
Stuffing	77
Waffles, pancakes	77
Watermelon	72-76
Carrots	65-76
White bread	75
French fries	75
Cheerios cereal	75
Corn bran cereal	75
Potatoes (boiled)	74
Bran Flakes cereal	74

Banana (over-ripe) 74
Graham crackers 74
Raisin Bran cereal 73
Potatoes (mashed) 73
Beer 73
Bagel (plain) 72
Saltine crackers, water crackers 72
Whole wheat bread 72
Millet 71
Cream of wheat cereal 71
Rice (regular, white) 70
Corn tortilla 70
English muffin 70
Shredded Wheat cereal 69
Corn meal 68
Wheat Thins crackers 68
Brown rice 68
Raisins 68
Baked beans (canned) 68
Grape-Nuts cereal .68
Gnocchi (potato pasta) 67
Life cereal 66
Oatmeal (quick cooking) 66
Pineapple 66
Banana 65
Melons 65
Couscous 65
Rye bread (regular) 64
Ice cream (regular; reduced fat varieties would
    have a higher rating) 64
Cola beverage 64
Orange juice 60
Popcorn 60
Pasta (regular white, refined) 60

Low Glycemic Index Foods

Eat More of These Foods to maintain healthy glucose levels!

GLYCEMIC INDEX

Celery, lettuce 0

Green vegetables, eggplant, onions, garlic, cauliflower, sprouts, radishes, etc. (fresh is lower than cooked) . .0-25

Eggs 10

Peanuts 10

Most meats and fish (unprocessed) 12

Yogurt (plain, unsweetened) 14

Soybeans 18

Fructose (fruit sugar) 22

Cherries 22

Plums 25

Grapefruit 25

Lentils (red) 25

Barley (pearled) 25

Milk (regular) 27

Kidney beans 27

Apricots, dried 30

Black beans 30

Kidney beans 30

Lentils (green) 30

Butter beans 31

Milk (skim) 32

Split peas 32

Strawberries, raspberries, blackberries (fresh) . . .32

Flax seeds 32

Chickpeas (garbanzo beans) 33

Vermicilli pasta 35

Pears 36

Tomatoes 38

Pinto beans 39

Navy beans 38

Yogurt (sweetened, regular fat) 38

Foods That Increase Risk of Diabetes

A study of more than 65,000 women by the Harvard School of Public Health showed that women who consumed the most sugar and the least amount of fiber ran two-and-a-half times the risk of developing diabetes as women who ate little sugar and lots of fiber.

Cereal fibers proved to be the most important kind of fiber lowering the risk of diabetes. Foods like cola beverages, white bread, crackers, white rice, french fries, desserts, and other highly refined foods low in fiber and vitamins and minerals increased the risk of diabetes.

Exercise

Consistent aerobic exercise can help keep your weight down and lower your risk of diabetes. Exercise conveys many other benefits: lowering the risk of heart disease and cancer, improving blood flow and muscle tone, and defusing stress.

When you exercise, your muscles work harder and consume glucose stores for fuel.

When the glucose stored in muscle runs low, glucose from the blood is withdrawn and burned. For someone who already has diabetes, this process eliminates a portion of the excess glucose that accumulates in the blood. As an added bonus, exercise seems to make muscles and other tissues more sensitive to insulin, so less of the hormone is needed to move glucose out of the blood and into muscle cells.

Diabetics should inform their doctor before starting an exercise program; exercise can cause a precipitous drop in blood glucose levels several hours after a workout.

Wholeness

...and as many as touched him were made **whole.** (Mark 6:56; emphasis added)

And Jesus answering said unto them, They that are **whole** *need not a physician; but they that are sick.* (Luke 5:31; emphasis added)

And he said unto her, Daughter, be of good comfort: thy faith hath made thee **whole***; go in peace.* (Luke 8:48; emphasis added)

The Greek translation of the Biblical word *health* is actually interchangeable with the word *wholeness* or *wellness*. Wholeness implies completeness. To be complete is to lack nothing.

Wholeness or wellness is comprised of three parts: Body, soul and spirit. The body refers to the physical. We must take care of the body providing it with proper rest, exercise and nutrition. The soul (sometimes referred to as our heart) involves our relationships to others, which includes our emotions, our memory and our will. The Bible instructs us to love one another. The spirit involves our relationship to God. God wants to have a personal and intimate relationship with us.

Wellness is interdependent upon all three aspects. We may have a good diet and even take supplements and yet still have health problems. The reason that health problems may not improve even after such physical improvements are made may lie in "illness" in the other two components required for wellness. If you are in disobedience (harboring unforgiveness, bitterness, etc.), God cannot bless you. If you have turned your back on God and do not have a personal relationship with Him, He cannot bless you. If you are not trusting God (living in fear – fear of man, fear of rejection, fear of abandonment, etc.) and are living a life filled with anxiety and stress, God cannot bless you.

Health Is a Blessing!

Deuteronomy 28 tells us that health is a blessing. In order for God to bless us we must be obedient to Him and we must have a personal relationship with Him. Deuteronomy 28 also tells us that health problems (disease) are a curse. Notice that the curse (disease) is conditional: The first word is *if.*

> *If thou wilt not observe to do all the words of this law that are written in this book,* that thou mayest fear this glorious and fearful name, THE LORD THY GOD; Then the LORD will make thy plagues wonderful, and the plagues *of thy seed* (your children) *even great plagues, and of long continuance, and sore **sicknesses**, and of long continuance. Moreover, **he will bring upon thee all the diseases** of Egypt, which thou wast afraid of; and they shall cleave unto thee.*
>
> ***Also every sickness, and every plague,*** *which [is] not written in the book of this law, them will*

*the LORD bring upon thee, until thou be destroyed... And the LORD shall scatter thee among all people, from the one end of the earth even unto the other; and there thou shalt serve other gods, which neither thou nor thy fathers have known, [even] wood and stone. And among these nations shalt thou find no ease, neither shall the sole of thy foot have rest: but the LORD shall give thee there a **trembling heart, and failing of eyes, and sorrow of mind:** And thy life shall hang in doubt before thee; and thou shalt fear day and night, and shalt have none assurance of thy life.* (Deuteronomy 28:58-66; emphasis added)

Deuteronomy 30 tells us that we have the power and ability to chose blessings or curses. He is telling us that we are in control of our health. If we are not in control, we need to get in control!

I have set before you life and death, blessings and cursing; therefore, choose life, that thou and thy seed (your children) may live; That thou mayest love the Lord thy God and that thou mayest obey His voice, and that thou mayest cleave unto Him, for He is the life, and the length of thy days. (Deuteronomy 30:19-20)

*If thou will diligently hearken to the voice of the LORD thy God, and will do that which is right in His sight, and will give ear to His commandments, and keep all His statutes, I will put none of these diseases upon thee, which I have brought upon the Egyptians: for **I am the LORD that healeth thee.*** (Exodus 15:26; emphasis added)

It is very important to realize that human responsibility is involved in much of the suffering that goes on. We suffer on our own account or because of what others have done to us. We should not blame God for the suffering that we bring upon ourselves or that others cause.

God is a Good God! It is His Desire to Heal Us!

Of course it is not God's perfect will that we suffer with illness. It is His will that we **do not get sick.** However, if disease enters our life, or the lives of our children, and we repent from our sin (bitterness, unforgiveness, fear, allowing stress and circumstances to rule our life, or not taking good care of the temple, etc.), God will restore us! This is a promise repeated many times in His Word. This is why Jesus came!

> *Jesus read from Isaiah (61:1), fulfilling the prophesy of His coming. The Spirit of the Lord is upon me, because he hath anointed me to preach the gospel to the poor; he hath sent me to heal the brokenhearted, to preach deliverance to the captives, and recovering of sight to the blind, to set at liberty them that are bruised.* (Luke 4:18)

> *Who forgives all thine iniquities; who heals* **all** *thy diseases!* (Psalm 103:3)

> *He was wounded for our transgressions, He was bruised for our iniquities: the chastisement of our peace was upon him; and with his stripes we are healed.* (Isaiah 53:5)

Because of Jesus' sacrifice on our behalf God will someday put an end to all suffering. *And I heard a loud voice from heaven saying, 'Behold, the tabernacle of God is with men and he will dwell with them, and they shall be his people, and God himself will be with them and be their God. And God shall wipe away every tear from their eyes; there shall be no more death, nor sorrow, nor crying; and there shall be no more pain, for the former things have passed away. Then he who sat on the throne said, 'Behold, I make all things new.* (Revelation 21:3-5)

Look how Jesus taught us to pray, *...Your kingdom come, your will be done, on earth as it is in heaven.* (Matthew 6:10) It is God's will that we ask for the things of heaven (no suffering) to come to us **now**, while we are still here. We do not have to wait for heaven to be whole!

Fearfully and Wonderfully Made

Our bodies are fearfully and wonderfully made (Psalm 139:14). Our bodies are designed to heal themselves. They are designed to maintain homeostasis or balance. This means if an invader like a bacteria or virus or even a toxin or cancerous cells is detected in the body, the body is designed to adjust accordingly to deal with the problem so that it does not create havoc.

Psychoneuroimmunolgly research reveals the physiological effects of stress on the body. In the 1950's Hans Selye, M.D., author of *The Stress of Life*, actually researched and revealed much of this information on the negative effects of cortisol (a hormone produced by the adrenal glands if there is any type of stress (physical or emotional) present). Some 50 years later the rest of the medical community is finally catching on.

According to Selye, life is largely a process of the

body's adaptation to the circumstances in which we exist. The secret of health and of peace lies in the successful adjustment to the ever-changing conditions of life.

Selye reports in detail how stress (in any form) affects the hypothalamous, the pituitary, the adrenal glands, the thyroid, the heart, digestion, appetite, reproductive glands and all aspects of the body. He explains how stress creates hormonal and chemical imbalances resulting in suppression of the immune system, inflammatory imbalances, sleep disturbances, and many other detrimental health effects. Anxiety and fear are forms of stress.

The very interesting missing component not discussed in Selye's book is the fact that many stressors such as fear and anxiety stem from our thoughts. We should be in control of our thoughts, not allowing our circumstances to rule us. The Bible tells us to take captive our every thought:

> *Casting down imaginations, and every high thing that exalteth itself against the knowledge of God, and bringing into captivity every thought to the obedience of Christ.* (2 Corinthians 10:5)

Our thoughts are what rule our emotions and cause us to have fear, anxiety, stress, depression, etc. If you think there is no reason to be afraid, then you will have no fear. If you are afraid that someone will criticize you for what you are wearing or what you said or you worry about what other people will think, you are living in fear. Your body does not know if your fear is from the fact that you are going to meet your mother-in-law for lunch or if a hungry lion is chasing you. The physiological response of the body is the same.

Fear (stress) causes the body to go into a heightened

state of alert. The hypothalamus produces neurotrans-mitters and hormones (such as cortisol) that increase blood pressure and heart rate, decrease digestive activi-ty, decrease your ability to sleep, and diminish the pro-duction of other neurotransmitters and hormones that rob us of our peace and joy (such as serotonin and dopamine). Lack of serotonin is a very common problem today. This is reflected in the very prevalent use of anti-depressant medications. Many of these are in the class referred to as SSRIs, which stands for selective serotonin reuptake inhibitors. They are designed to continually recycle the small amount of serotonin that you are pro-ducing. This reminds me of never changing the oil in your car; it's no wonder that they have so many side effects, which get worse the longer the medication is taken.

If you are depressed, you need to change your thoughts. The Bible tells us we are to get our joy from the Lord (Philippians 3:1) and **not** from our circum-stances. Because so many people do focus on their cir-cumstances, it is no surprise that so many are depressed and anxious.

Set your affection on things above, not on things on the earth. (Colossians 3:2)

If your thoughts cause you to feel fear and anxiety, you need to change your thoughts. A mature person is not double-minded (unstable) but has a sound mind. It is your choice whether you allow your circumstances to mature you or to put you into a state of continual fear and anxiety.

Fear is not just an emotion; the Bible calls fear an evil spirit. Evil spirits can be rejected and cast off.

For God did not give you a spirit of fear; but of power,
of love, and of a sound mind. (2 Timothy 1:7)

The negative effect that fear and stress have on our body is one of the reasons we need to be in control of our thoughts. Why are you allowing yourself to become stressed? Life will be filled with stressful events. Stress does not go away after we reach a certain age or after we get married or have children or get divorced or get the car fixed or get a better job or move into a bigger house and on and on. We are not to allow these events or circumstances to rule us. We should not base our joy upon our circumstances. If we do we will always be disappointed, because life is not without trials. There will be consequences because, according to the Word and now confirmed by medical science, our health will suffer. We will never have true joy or peace because it will only be fleeting and will fade as soon as the next trying circumstance comes our way. We are not to be double-minded or unstable. An unstable person sways according to his or her circumstances.

Do not be wise in your own eyes; fear the LORD and shun evil. This will bring health to your body and nourishment to your bones. (Proverbs 3:7-8)

Because it is our choice whether we receive blessing or curses, we must decide which one to choose.

Pastor Henry Wright, author of the book, *A More Excellent Way: A Teaching on the Spiritual Roots of Disease*, states that all disease is a result of separation on some level:

1. Separation from God, His Word, and His love. For example, from unrepentive sin, rebellion, rejection of God, fear, etc.

2. Separation from yourself. For example, not accepting yourself, not loving yourself (self-rejection), feeling guilt and condemnation. We often do not realize that self-rejection in its various forms is sin. We were created in God's image.

> So God created man in his [own] image, in the image of God created he him; male and female created he them... And God saw every thing that he had made, and, behold, it was very good. (Genesis 1:27, 31)

3. Separation from others. For example, unforgiveness, envy, jealousy, broken relationships, lack of nurturing, lack of love, abuse, perfectionism, etc.

Matthew 6:15 shows how our unforgiveness of others is a stumbling block to our healing: *But if forgive not men their trespasses, neither will your Father forgive your trespasses,*

Many of you are reading this book because either you or a loved one is diabetic or you have been told you are on your way to developing diabetes. For those who developed diabetes at a young age, the idea of having a spiritual root for your health problems may be very difficult to understand. You are probably thinking, "This started at age four, if it is our choice, how could God hold a four-year-old responsible?" I am not saying it is entirely your fault. Many things are passed on through the generations. It may be a generational curse.

Thou shalt not bow down thyself to them, nor serve

them: for I the LORD thy God am a jealous God, vis-
iting the iniquity of the fathers upon the children
unto the third and fourth generation of them that
hate me; And showing mercy unto thousands of
them that love me, and keep my commandments.
(Exodus 20:5-6)

What the medical community refers to as hereditary, the Bible calls a generational curse. Through Christ and our obedience, we have the ability to break off generational curses. Because of our lack of knowledge, many of us did not even realize there was such a thing as a generational curse. This is no excuse, Hosea 4:6 tells us *My people are destroyed for lack of knowledge.* It is our own responsibility to get into the Word and find out these things!

Spiritual Roots

The root of a disease simply refers to the cause. What is causing the body to malfunction? The three types of root to consider for wellness are:

1. Body (the physical)

2. Soul (relationship with others, which includes our emotions, thoughts, etc.)

3. Spirit (relationship with God)

Many ask, if this health problem is a curse, why would God curse me? *As the bird by wandering, as the swallow by flying, so the curse causeless shall not come.* (Proverbs 26:2) This is the same principal as "we reap what we sow."

Suffering entered into God's universe as a result of sin. This occurred when Adam and Eve disobeyed God at the prompting of the devil. Because of their disobedience God pronounced judgment upon them. This included that they would suffer in this life.

To the woman he said: *I will greatly multiply your sorrow and your conception; in pain you shall bring forth children; your desire shall be for your husband, and he shall rule over you.*

To Adam he said: *Cursed is the ground for your sake; in toil you shall eat of it all the days of your life. Both thorns and thistles it shall bring forth for you, and you shall eat the herb of the field. In the sweat of your face you shall eat bread till you return to the ground, for out of it you were taken; for dust you are, and to dust you shall return.* (Genesis 3:16-19)

Specific examples of spiritual roots the Bible points out include: *A sound heart is the life of the flesh: but envy the rottenness of the bones* (Proverbs 14:30) and *A merry heart doeth good like a medicine: but a broken spirit drieth the bones.* (Proverbs 17:22)

We are not just talking about osteoporosis here, the bones are especially significant to our overall health and the integrity of the immune system because it is in the bone marrow that we produce our blood cells.

Autoimmune Disease Roots

Autoimmune diseases include lupus, rheumatoid arthritis, multiple sclerosis (MS), Type I diabetes. In these diseases the body attacks itself, destroying healthy cells. In Type I diabetes, the body attacks the pancreas interfering with its ability to produce insulin. In MS the body destroys the myelin sheath (which is the protective coating on the nerves) interfering with movement. In rheumatoid arthritis, the connective tissue between the joints is destroyed. In allergies and asthma, white blood cells are, in a sense, overreactive to things that the body does not need to be protected from, like pollen or certain foods. This produces many unpleasant symptoms such as bronchial constriction, runny nose or skin rashes.

Long-term fear is a cause of many health problems, autoimmune problems in particular. Autoimmune problems are also often associated with self-hatred and self-rejection. While the immune system is designed to protect our health, in autoimmune diseases, the body instead attacks itself (or an otherwise harmless substance in the case of allergies). Medical science has no known root causes for most autoimmune diseases.

Pastor Henry Wright, in *A More Excellent Way – A Teaching on the Spiritual Roots of Disease*, states that the spiritual root behind Type I diabetes (an auto-immune disease) is extreme self-rejection and self-hatred coupled with guilt. He reports many victorious physical healings in conjunction with healing of the spiritual woundedness.

Self-rejection can result from many things. Lack of proper parenting from two parents is a major cause. If you consider the divorce rates today, the number of people with diabetes is not that surprising. If one of your parents left when you were young, this often leaves long-term, deep-rooted rejection woundings. A child often (and sometimes unknowingly) blames himself, thinking it was his fault. This is guilt. This is a lie from the enemy.

The lack of fathering (including fathers who do not know **how** to father) is one of the nation's biggest problems today. God created families with two parents because, in His divine wisdom, He knew that this is what children needed.

What if abortion was considered or the pregnancy was unplanned or unwanted? This is rejection of a very high magnitude. The child (even the unborn) can sense this, and the enemy will use it to attack at any given opportunity.

Self-rejection is a huge problem today. So many people feel unworthy, unwanted, and unhappy with themselves. The false expectations of society, advertising and media, etc., compound the situation and it is no wonder that so many feel inadequate for some reason. At some time in your life you started believing the lies that were told to you or you may even tell yourself (you are not good enough, you are not going to amount to anything, you are a loser, you are not as attractive or gifted or skilled as other people, etc.). If you have fallen for these lies, and believe they are true, you need to **change your thinking!** These are lies from the enemy who is using others to make you feel this way. You need to realize who is headed for a lake of fire and who is a new creature in Christ! When we accept Christ as our personal savior, *we become a new creature: old things are passed away; behold, all things are become new.* (2 Corinthians 5:17)

The Bible teaches that every one of us is very special. Jesus Christ, God the Son, came down from heavens glory just to die on our behalf. The Bible says, when we were still powerless, Christ died for the ungodly. Very rarely will anyone die for a righteous man, though for a good man someone might possibly dare to die. But God demonstrates his own love for us in this: *While we were still sinners, Christ died for us.* (Romans 5: 6-8)

> Pastor Wright says, *In many cases that we have ministered to in the past 10 years, we've found that there was a direct rejection by a father and sometimes, a husband or a man in general.*

He also writes that diabetes can be inherited because fear can be passed from one generation to the next and an unloving spirit can also be passed on. He also writes that a broken heart can also be the cause.

Whenever there is abuse, there is victimization and rejection. Often, when one is repeatedly told "you are a failure" or some other negative comment, the individual will eventually begin to believe it. In our desire to be loved and accepted, when we are not, we may feel it is because of a fault of our own. Don't fall for it! Each one of us was created in the image of God and everything that God created is very good!

Type II Diabetes Root

Adult-onset diabetes is believed to have a more physical root from improper care of the body. Obesity and overeating and poor dietary habits (too many refined foods) are major risk factors associated with Type II onset.

Turning to food for comfort instead of God can actually be considered a form of idolatry. Most people do not think of addiction to food as sin, but it definitely is. Overeating accompanies this behavior, as food will never fill the "God-shaped" void that God has put within us. We will never truly be satisfied by anything other than God.

Most addictions are rooted in a need for love (that can only be cured by accepting the love that God has for us!)

101

This is the only way to "fill" the void.

Science has confirmed that Type II diabetes is preventable and correctable through proper diet. This simply verifies God's promises. If we repent (turn from our evil ways), He will restore us!

> Therefore I will judge you, O house of Israel, every one according to his ways, saith the Lord GOD. Repent, and turn [yourselves] from all your transgressions; so iniquity shall not be your ruin. (Ezekiel 18:30)

> If my people, which are called by my name, shall humble themselves, and pray, and seek my face, and turn from their wicked ways; then will I hear from heaven, and will forgive their sin, and will heal their land. (2 Chronicles 7:14)

Sin is *Not* the Cause of *All* Disease!

Remember, it may not **always** be possible to know the root cause of a particular physical or mental illness. The Bible also tells us that sin is not the cause of all disease. *And his disciples asked him, saying, Master, who did sin, this man, or his parents, that he was born blind? Jesus answered, Neither hath this man sinned, nor his parents: but that the works of God should be made manifest in him.* (John 9:2-3)

It is wise to prayerfully consider the possibility of the three areas (body, soul, spirit) discussed in this book to reveal the root. Because we know *the curse causeless shall not come* (Proverbs 26:2), we know there is a reason when illness enters our life. When the root is revealed, you will then know how to deal with it and healing can begin!

Conclusions... in Prayer

It is God's Desire to Heal Us! We have examined many examples from God's Word of promises that He not only forgives us for our sin, but He also heals us from all diseases. We need to believe and claim these promises He makes to us!

Don't forget, there is power in prayer! To determine what changes to make after reading the information in this book, ask God for guidance. Search your heart for things that God wants to free from you from (stress, fears, anxiety, unforgiveness, bitterness, self-rejection, guilt, etc.) and repent. Ask God to reveal to you what changes in all areas of wellness need to be made in your life so that you can be healed.

For more information on this subject, I suggest reading my book, *God Wants You Well!* and Pastor Henry Wrights book, *A More Excellent Way - A Teaching on the Spiritual Roots of Disease.*

It does not matter what your health problems are or how long you have had them, all people can be free of sickness and disease. The Bible teaches us that Jesus came not only to preach the good news to the poor, but to **heal the brokenhearted** and to **set the captives free!** Don't be held captive to the lies of the enemy! Be well!

Who forgives all thine iniquities; who heals __all__ thy diseases! (Psalms 103:3)

103

Bibliography

Anderson RA. Chromium in the prevention and control of diabetes. Diabetes Metab 2000 Feb;26(1):22-7

Anderson RA, Roussel AM, Zouari N, Mahjoub S, Matheau JM, Kerkeni A. Potential antioxidant effects of zinc and chromium supplementation in people with type 2 diabetes mellitus. J Am Coll Nutr 2001 Jun;20(3):212-8.

Anderson RA, Cheng N, Bryden NA, Polansky MM, Cheng N, Chi J, Feng J. Elevated intakes of supplemental chromium improve glucose and insulin variables in individuals with type 2 diabetes. Diabetes. 1997 Nov;46(11):1786-91.

Anderson JW, Konz EC, Jenkins DJ. Health advantages and disadvantages of weight-reducing diets: a computer analysis and critical review. J Am Coll Nutr 2000 Oct;19(5):578-90.

Bahijiri SM, Mira SA, Mufti AM, Ajabnoor MA. The effects of inorganic chromium and brewer's yeast supplementation on glucose tolerance, serum lipids and drug dosage in individuals with type 2 diabetes.Saudi Med J 2000 Sep;21(9):831-7

Ben-Aryeh H, et al. Oral health and salivary composition in diabetic patients. J Diabetes Complications. 1993 Jan-Mar;7(1):57-62.

Bereket A; Lang CH; Wilson TA; Alterations in the growth hormone-insulin-like growth factor axis in insulin dependent diabetes mellitus. Horm Metab Res 1999 Feb-Mar;31(2-3):172-81.

Brandao-Neto J, Silva CA, Shuhama T, Silva JA, Oba L; Renal handling of zinc in insulin-dependent diabetes mellitus patients. Biometals 2001 Mar;14(1):75-80.

Chan P, Tomlinson B, Chen YJ, Liu JC, Hsieh MH, Cheng JT. A double-blind placebo-controlled study of the effectiveness and tolerability of oral stevioside in human hypertension. Br J Clin Pharmacol 2000 Sep;50(3):215-20.

Curi R, Alvarez M, Bazotte RB, et al. Effect of Stevia rebaudiana on glucose tolerance in normal adult humans. Braz J Med Biol Res 1986;19(6):771–74.

Dunger DB; Acerini CL; IGF-I and diabetes in adolescence. Diabetes Metab 1998 Apr;24(2):101-7.

Eriksson JG, Forsen TJ, Mortensen SA, Rohde M. The effect of coenzyme Q10 administration on metabolic control in patients with type 2 diabetes mellitus. Biofactors 1999;9(2-4):315-8.

Florkowski CM, Scott RS, Coope PA, Moir CL;.Predictors of mortality from type 2 diabetes mellitus in Canterbury, New Zealand; a ten-year cohort study. Diabetes Res Clin Pract. 2001 Aug;53(2):113-20.

Gatling W, Guzder RN, Turnbull JC, Budd S, Mullee MA. The Poole Diabetes Study: how many cases of Type 2 diabetes are diagnosed each year during normal health care in a defined community? Diabetes Res Clin Pract. 2001 Aug;53(2):107-12.

Goke B; Fehmann HC; Insulin and insulin-like growth factor-I: their role as risk factors in the development of diabetic cardiovascular disease. Diabetes Res Clin Pract 1996 Feb;30 Suppl:93-106.

Gupta R, Garg VK, Mathur DK, Goyal RK. Oral zinc therapy in diabetic neuropathy. Dept. of Medicine, JLN Medical College and Associated Group of Hospital, Ajmer, Rajasthan-305 001. J Assoc Physicians India 1998 Nov;46(11):939-42.

Haglund B, Ryckenberg K, Selinus O, Dahlquist G.; Evidence of a relationship between childhood-onset Type I diabetes and low groundwater concentration of zinc. Centre for Epidemiology, National Board of Social Welfare, Stockholm, Sweden. Diabetes Care 1996 Aug;19(8):873-5.

Henriksen JE, Andersen CB, Hother-Nielsen O, Vaag A, Mortensen SA, Beck-Nielsen H. Impact of ubiquinone (coenzyme Q10) treatment on glycemic control, insulin requirement and well-being in patients with Type 1 diabetes mellitus. Diabet Med 1999 Apr;16(4):312-8.

Hermansen K, Sondergaard M, Hoie L, Carstensen M, Brock B.; Beneficial effects of a soy-based dietary supplement on lipid levels and cardiovascular risk markers in type 2 diabetic subjects. Diabetes Care. 2001 Feb;24(2):228-33.

Hu FB, van Dam RM, Liu S., Diet and risk of Type II diabetes: the role of types of fat and carbohydrate.Nutr. 2001 Jun;73(6):1001-2.

Jeppesen PB, Gregersen S, Poulsen CR, Hermansen K.; Stevioside acts directly on pancreatic beta cells to secrete insulin: actions independent of cyclic adenosine monophosphate and adenosine triphosphate-sensitive K+-channel activity. Metabolism 2000 Feb;49(2):208-14.

Karahan SC, Deger O, Orem A, Ucar F, Erem C, Alver A, Onder E; The effects of impaired trace element status on polymorphonuclear leukocyte activation in the development of vascular complications in type 2 diabetes mellitus. Dep. of Biochemistry, Faculty of Medicine, KTU, Trabzon, Turkey. Clin Chem Lab Med 2001 Feb;39(2):109-15.

Kavet R, Nauss KM.; The toxicity of inhaled methanol vapors. Crit Rev Toxicol. 1990;21(1):21-50. Review. PMID: 2264926

Kelly GS. Insulin resistance: lifestyle and nutritional interventions. Altern Med Rev 2000.Apr;5(2):109-32.

Kilic F., Packer. L., Trevethick, J.R. Modeling corticol cataracogenesis 17: Invitro effect of a-Lipoic Acid on glucose-induced lens membrane damage, a model of diabetic cataractogenesis Exp. Eye Res (1994).

Kilic F; Handelman GJ; Serbinova E; Packer L; Trevithick JR; Modelling cortical cataractogenesis 17: in vitro effect of a-a-Lipoic Acid on glucose-induced lens membrane damage, a model of diabetic cataractogenesis. Dept. of Biochemistry, University of Western Ontario, London, Canada. Biochem Mol Biol Int 1995 Oct;37(2):361-70.

Kimura K.; Role of essential trace elements in the disturbance of carbohydrate metabolism]. Department of Biochemistry, Faculty of Medicine, Tottori University.1: Nippon Rinsho 1996 Jan;54(1):79-84.

Kruse-Jarres JD, Rukgauer M.; Trace elements in diabetes mellitus. Peculiarities and clinical validity of determinations in blood cells. .Katharinenhospital, Institute of Clinical Chemistry and Laboratory Medicine, Stuttgart, Germany. J Trace Elem Med Biol 2000 Apr;14(1):21-7.

Lacka B; Grzeszczak W; Genetic aspects of diabetic retinopathy. Wiad Lek 1998;51 Suppl 2:24-9.

Larsen HN, Rasmussen OW, Rasmussen PH, Alstrup KK, Biswas SK, Tetens I, Thilsted SH, Hermansen K. Glycemic index of parboiled rice depends on the severity of processing: study in type 2 diabetic subjects. Eur J Clin Nutr. 2000 May;54(5):380-5.

Leung AY, Foster S. Encyclopedia of Common Natural Ingredients Used in Foods, Drugs, and Cosmetics, 2d ed. New York: John Wiley & Sons, 1996, 478–80.

Liu S, Manson JE, Stampfer MJ, et al; A prospective study of whole-grain intake and risk of type 2 diabetes mellitus in US women. Brigham and Women's Hospital, Harvard Medical School, Boston, Am J Public Health 2000 Sep;90(9):1409-15.

Low, P.A., K. Nickander, L.D. Schmelzer, M. Kihara, M. Nagamatsu & H. Tritschler; Experimental Diabetic Neuropathy: Idcremia, Oxidative Stress, and Neuroprotection, Mayo Fountaion and Asta Medica Dresdan, Germany Oxidants and Antioxidants in Biology, Oxygen Club of California, Annual Meeting, March 1995.

Lupia E; Elliot SJ; Lenz O; Zheng F; Hattori M; Striker GE; Striker LJ; GF-1 decreases collagen degradation in diabetic NOD mesangial cells: implications for diabetic nephropathy. University of Miami School of Medicine, Florida. Diabetes 1999 Aug;48(8):1638-44.

Manzella D, Barbieri M, Ragno E, Paolisso G.; Chronic administration of pharmacologic doses of vitamin E improves the cardiac autonomic nervous system in patients with type 2 diabetes. Am J Clin Nutr 2001 Jun;73(6):1052-7.

McCarty MF. Can correction of sub-optimal coenzyme Q status improve beta-cell function in type II diabetics? Med Hypotheses 1999 May;52(5):397-400.

McCarty MF. Toward practical prevention of type 2 diabetes. Med Hypotheses 2000 May;54(5):786-93

McDonnell MG.; Archbold GP; Plasma ubiquinol/cholesterol ratios in patients with hyperlipidaemia, those with diabetes mellitus and in patients requiring dialysis. Belfast City Hospital, N. Ireland, UK. Clin Chim Acta 1996 Sep 30;253(1-2):117-26.

Melis MS. A crude extract of Stevia rebaudiana increases the renal plasma flow of normal and hypertensive rats. Braz J Med Biol Res1996;29(5):669–75.

Monte, W.C."Aspartame: Methanol and the Public Health" Journal of Applied Nutrition, 1984 36(1): 42-53.

Nagamatsu. M, Nickander, K.K, Schmelzer, J.D., Raya, A., Wittrock, D.A., Tritschler, H., Low, P.A.; "Lipoic Acid improves nerve blood flow, reduces oxidative stress, and improves distal nerve conduction in experimental diabetic neuropathy." Diabetes Care 1995 Aug;18(8):1160-7.

Packer, L.; Antioxidant properties of a-Lipoic Acid and its therapeutic effects in prevention of diabetes complications and cataracts. Ann N Y Acad Sci 1994 Nov 17;738:257-64

Pick ME, Hawrysh ZJ, Gee MI, Toth E, Garg ML, Hardin RT.; Oat bran concentrate bread products improve long-term control of diabetes: a pilot ,,study. Department of Agricultural, Food and Nutritional Science, University of Alberta, Edmonton, Canada. J Am Diet Assoc 1996 Dec;96(12):1254-61.

Posner HS. Biohazards of methanol in proposed new uses. J Toxicol Environ Health. 1975 Sep;1(1):153-71. Review.

Raman A, Lau C. Anti-diabetic properties and phytochemistry of Momordica charantia L (Curcurbitaceae). Phytomed Res 1996; 2:349-62.

Rasmussen O, Winther E, Hermansen K; Postprandial glucose and insulin responses to rolled oats ingested raw, cooked or as a mixture with raisins in normal subjects and type 2 diabetic patients.Diabet Med 1989 May-Jun;6(4):337-41

Rauscher FM, Sanders RA, Watkins JB 3rd. Effects of coenzyme Q10 treatment on antioxidant pathways in normal and streptozotocin-induced diabetic rats.J Biochem Mol Toxicol 2001;15(1):41-6.

Roe O. Species differences in methanol poisoning. Crit Rev Toxicol. 1982 Oct;10(4):275-86. Review.

Salmeron J, Hu FB, Manson JE, Stampfer MJ, Colditz GA, Rimm EB, Willett WC. Dietary fat intake and risk of type 2 diabetes in women.Am J Clin Nutr 2001 Jun;73(6):1019-26.

Salonen, J, et al; Increased risk of noninsulin-dependent diabetes mellitus at low plasma Vitamin E concentrations. A 3 year follow-up study in men. BMJ,1995, 28;311:1124-7.

Segev Y; Landau D; et al; Growth hormone receptor antagonism prevents early renal changes in nonobese diabetic mice. J Am Soc Nephrol 1999 Nov;10(11):2374-81.

Singh RB, Niaz MA, Rastogi SS, Bajaj S, Gaoli Z, Shoumin Z.; Current zinc intake and risk of diabetes and coronary artery disease and factors associated with insulin resistance in rural and urban populations of North India. Center of Nutrition and Heart Research Laboratory, Medical Hospital and Research Center, Moradabad, India. J Am Coll Nutr 1998 Dec;17(6):564-70. comment in J Am Coll Nutr. 1998 Dec;17(6):542-3.

Simon SF, Taylor CG.; Dietary zinc supplementation attenuates hyperglycemia in db/db mice. Department of Food and Nutrition, University of Manitoba, Winnipeg, Canada. Exp Biol Med (Maywood) 2001 Jan;226(1):43-51.

Stoddard, Mary Nash, 1995. Conversations between Mary Nash Stoddard of the Aspartame Consumer Safety Network and Mark D. Gold. and Mission Possible

1994. Compiled by researchers, physicians, and artificial sweetner experts for Mission Possible, a group dedicated to warning consumers about aspartame. Mission Possible, 9270 River Club Pkwy, Duluth, Georgia 30155.

Strodter, D.; Lehmann, E.; Lehmann, U.; Tritschler, H.J.; Bretzel RG; The influence of thioctic acid on metabolism and function of the diabetic heart. Medical Clinic III, University of Giessen, Germany. Diabetes Res Clin Pract 1995 Jul;29(1):19-26.

Studt,. J.; Heuer, L.J.; Diabetic autonomic neuropathy of the heart and its treatment with thioctic acid Dtsch Z Verdau Stoffwechselkr 1984;44(4): 173-80.

Suzuki YJ, Mizuno M, Tritschler HJ, Packer L. Redox regulation of NF-kappa B DNA binding activity by dihydrolipoate. Biochem Mol Biol Int. 1995 Jun;36(2):241-6.

Suzuki YJ, Tsuchiya M, Packer L. Lipoate prevents glucose-induced protein modifications. Free Radic Res Commun. 1992;17(3):211-7.

Thomas, Frank et al.: Increased weight gain, nitrogen retention and muscle protein zynthesis following treatment of diabetic rats with IGF-I anddes 1-3 (IGF-I). BlochemJ. 1991,276: 547- 554- 547.

Thomsen C, Rasmussen O, Christiansen C, Pedersen E, Vesterlund M, Storm H, Ingerslev J, Hermansen K.; Comparison of the effects of a monounsaturated fat diet and a high carbohydrate diet on cardiovascular risk factors in first degree relatives to type-2 diabetic subjects. Eur J Clin Nutr. 1999 Oct;53(10):818-23.

Trefz F, de Sonneville L, Matthis P, Benninger C, Lanz-Englert B, Bickel H. Neuropsychological and biochemical investigations in heterozygotes for phenylketonuria during ingestion of high dose aspartame (a sweetener containing phenylalanine). Hum Genet 1994 Apr;93(4):369-74.

Tephly TR;. Comments on the purported generation of formaldehyde and adduct formation from the sweetener aspartame. Life Sci. 1999;65(13):PL157-60.

Trevithick, J.R., F. Kilic, G.J Handelman, E. Serbinow & L. Packer "In Vitro Effect of a-Lipoic Acid on Glucose-induced Lens membrane damage, a model of Diabetic Cataractgenesis" University of Western Ontario, London, Ontario, and University of California, Berkley, *Oxidants and Antioxidants in Biology,* Oxygen Club of California, Annual Meeting, March 1995.

Tritschler, P. HJ, Wolff, S.P., Thiotic (lipoic) acid: a therapeutic metal-chelating antioxidant? Biochem Pharmacol 1995 Jun 29;50(1):123-6.

Trocho C, Pardo R, Rafecas I, Virgili J, Remesar X, Fernandez-Lopez JA, Alemany M. Formaldehyde derived from dietary aspartame binds to tissue components in vivo. Life Sci. 1998;63(5):337-49.

US FDA, U.S. Court of Appeals for the District of Columbia Circuit, No. 84-1153 Community Nutrition Institute and Dr. Woodrow Monte v. Dr. Mark Novitch, Acting Commissioner, US FDA (9/24/85).

Van den Eeden SK, Koepsell TD, Longstreth WT Jr, van Belle G, Daling JR, McKnight B.; Aspartame ingestion and headaches: a randomized crossover trial. Department of Epidemiology, School of Public Health and Community Medicine, University of Washington, Seattle 98195. Neurology 1994 Oct;44(10):1787-93.

Wang SR, Chase HP, Garg SK, Hoops SL, Harris MA.; The effect of sugar cereal with and without a mixed meal on glycemic response in children with diabetes. Barbara Davis Center for Childhood Diabetes, Department of Pediatrics, University of Colorado Health, Sciences Center, Denver. J Pediatr Gastroenterol Nutr 1991 Aug;13(2):155-60.

Wright, Henry. A More Excellent Way - A Teaching on the Spiritual Roots of Disease. Pleasant Valley Publications, Thomaston, GA . 800-453-5775. (2000).

Wursch P, Pi-Sunyer FX. The role of viscous soluble fiber in the metabolic control of diabetes. A review with special emphasis on cereals rich in beta-glucan.Nestle Research Centre, Lausanne, Switzerland. Diabetes Care 1997 Nov;20(11):1774-80.

Index

ABOUT THE AUTHOR

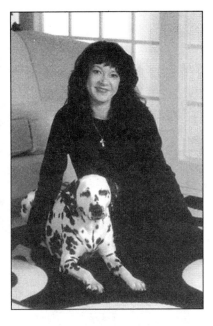

Beth M. Ley, Ph.D., has been a science writer specializing in health and nutrition since 1988 and has written many health-related books, including the best sellers, ***DHEA: Unlocking the Secrets to the Fountain of Youth*** and ***MSM: On Our Way Back to Health With Sulfur.*** She wrote her own undergraduate degree program and graduated in Scientific and Technical Writing from North Dakota State University in 1987 (combination of Zoology and Journalism). Beth has her masters (1998) and doctoral degrees (1999) in Nutrition.

Beth does nutrition and wellness counseling at The Wellness Center in Detroit Lakes, MN, and speaks on nutrition, health and divine healing locally and nationwide. She is a weekly speaker at Strawberry Lake Christian Retreat, Ogema, MN.

Beth lives in the Minnesota lakes country. She is dedicated to God and to spreading the health message. She enjoys nature and spending time with her dalmatian, KC.

Memberships: American Academy of Anti-aging, New York Academy of Sciences, Oxygen Society and Resurrection Apostolic International Network (RAIN), Gospel Crusade.

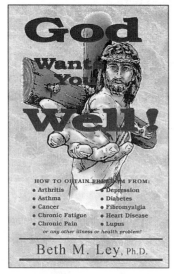
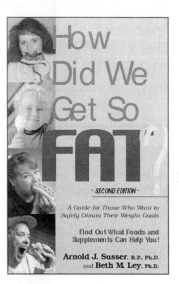

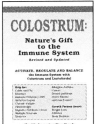
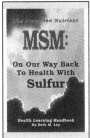
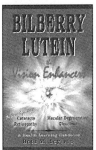
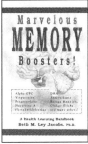
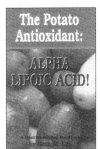
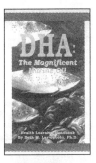

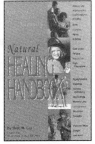